ERRATUM

Unfortunately, the wrong image was printed as Figure 1.2.

Please substitute the figure below for the one printed on page 8.

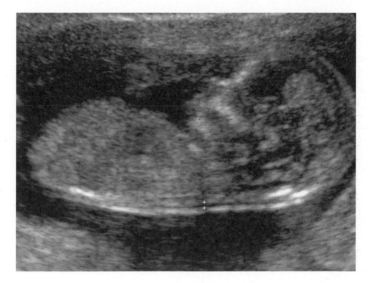

Figure 1.2 Nuchal translucency measurement, indicated by the calipers

Fetal Medicine
for the
MRCOG
and Beyond

Published titles in the MRCOG and Beyond series

Antenatal Disorders for the MRCOG and Beyond
by Andrew Thomson and Ian Greer

Gynaecological and Obstetric Pathology for the MRCOG
*by Harold Fox and C. Hilary Buckley, with a chapter on Cervical Cytology
by Dulcie V. Coleman*

Intrapartum Care for the MRCOG and beyond *by Thomas F. Baskett and
Sabaratnam Arulkumaran, with a chapter on Neonatal Resuscitation by John
McIntyre and a chapter on Perinatal Loss by Carolyn Basak*

Management of Infertility for the MRCOG and Beyond
by Allan A. Templeton et al.

Menopause for the MRCOG and Beyond *by Margaret Rees*

Menstrual Problems for the MRCOG *by Mary Ann Lumsden,
Jane Norman and Hilary Critchley*

Neonatology for the MRCOG *by Peter Dear and Simon Newell*

The MRCOG: A Guide to the Examination *by Ian Johnson et al.*

Forthcoming titles in the series

Early Pregnancy Issues

Gynaecological Oncology

Gynaecological Urology

Molecular Medicine

Reproductive Endocrinology

Fetal Medicine for the MRCOG and beyond

Alan Cameron MD MRCOG
Fetal Medicine Specialist,
The Queen Mother's Hospital, Yorkhill, Glasgow G3 8SJ, UK

Janet Brennand MD MRCOG
Consultant in Fetal and Maternal Medicine,
The Queen Mother's Hospital, Yorkhill, Glasgow G3 8SJ, UK

Lena Macara MD MRCOG
Consultant Obstetrician and Gynaecologist,
The Queen Mother's Hospital, Yorkhill, Glasgow G3 8SJ, UK

Peter Milton MD FRCOG
Consultant Obstetrician and Gynaecologist,
Addenbrooke's and Rosie Maternity Hospital,
Robinson Way, Cambridge CB2 2SW, UK

RCOG Press

First published 2002

© The Royal College of Obstetricians and Gynaecologists

ISBN 1-900364-74-3

Published by the **RCOG Press** at
The Royal College of Obstetricians and Gynaecologists
27 Sussex Place, Regent's Park
London NW1 4RG

Registered charity no. 213280

Cover illustration: The fetal medicine team at The Queen Mother's Hospital, Glasgow, performing an intravascular intrauterine transfusion

Cover photograph by Catherine Clark, Medical Illustration Department, Yorkhill

RCOG Editor: Jane Moody

Designed by Tony Crowley

Printed by Cambrian Printers, Llanbadarn Road, Aberystwyth, Ceredigion SY23 3TN

Acknowledgements
The authors would like to acknowledge the help and assistance of the Medical Illustration Department, Yorkhill NHS Trust, with particular thanks to Catherine Clark, who devoted many hours to the photographs and illustrations for this book. The authors would also like to thank the staff and patients of the Ultrasound Department at The Queen Mother's Hospital, without whose cooperation this work could not be performed. Finally, we would like to acknowledge Ian Donald's vision, which has inspired us all.

Contents

Plates   ii

Preface   iii

Abbreviations   iv

1   Screening for chromosomal abnormalities   1
Janet Brennand

2   Prenatal diagnostic techniques   13
Peter Milton

3   The routine anomaly scan   27
Lena Macara

4   Fetal structural abnormalities   41
Janet Brennand

5   Fetal therapy   55
Alan Cameron

6   Prenatal diagnosis and management of   87
non-immune hydrops fetalis
Alan Cameron

7   Termination of pregnancy for   101
fetal abnormality
Alan Cameron

8   Intrauterine growth restriction   109
Lena Macara

9   Twin pregnancy   123
Lena Macara

Index   139

Plates

PLATE 1   **Figure 4.2**   Open spina bifida
             Figure 4.4   Occipital encephalocele

PLATE 2   **Figure 4.5**   Gastroschisis: the anterior abdominal wall
                              defect is to the right of the umbilical cord
             Figure 5.4b Hydrops fetalis

PLATE 3   **Figure 5.6a** Measurement of cerebral artery peak systolic
                              velocity: Doppler ultrasound
             Figure 5.7a Intravascular transfusion

PLATE 4   **Figure 5.12** A fetus with 'prune belly' syndrome
             Figure 5.15 Neonate with pleuroamniotic shunt in place

PLATE 5   **Figure 5.16** Twin-to-twin transfusion syndrome;
                              donor left, recipient right
             Figure 5.17 Surviving fetuses of twin-to-twin transfusion
                              syndrome; donor left, recipient right

PLATE 6   **Figure 6.1** Stillborn hydropic neonate
             Figure 6.6 Human parvovirus B19

PLATE 7   **Figure 6.7** Slapped cheek syndrome
             Figure 6.8 Hydropic intrauterine death due to
                              parvovirus B19

PLATE 8   **Figure 8.2** A vascular cast of placental cotyledon: the
                              vessels supplying a cotyledon were injected
                              with plastic to form a mould of the vessel
                              network; once set the surrounding placental
                              tissue was digested with acid solution,
                              leaving the plastic mould of the vessels
                              within the villi; the extensive network of
                              vessels can be clearly seen and can then be
                              examined by scanning microscopy

Preface

Is the baby going to be normal? This is the question at the forefront of every prospective parent's mind. Although no single investigation or indeed battery of parental investigations can provide total reassurance with regard to the normality or wellbeing of any fetus, there have been major advances in the field of fetal medicine over the past few decades. All of these advances are dependent upon diagnostic ultrasound, which has revolutionised obstetric practice since its introduction by Professor Ian Donald half a century ago. It is thus particularly fitting that the contributions to this extremely important addition to the *MRCOG and Beyond* series emanate from The Queen Mother's Hospital in Glasgow, where ultrasound was introduced and developed.

A working knowledge of fetal medicine is essential for both aspiring specialists in obstetrics and gynaecology and established practitioners and this book comprehensively covers the whole field, with contributions relating not only to diagnostic techniques but also, most importantly, to the management of fetal abnormality following diagnosis. It will undoubtedly be a most valuable addition to the literature relating to this extremely exciting and rapidly advancing field of obstetric practice.

Peter Milton
June 2002

Abbreviations

α-FP	alphafetoprotein
bpm	beats per minute
CAH	congenital adrenal hyperplasia
CCAM	congenital cystic adenomatoid malformation of the lung
CHD	congenital heart disease
CMV	cytomegalovirus
COX	cyclo-oxygenase
CTG	cardiotocography
CVS	chorionic villus sampling
D&E	dilatation and evacuation
FFN	fetal fibronectin
FISH	fluorescence *in situ* hybridisation
FMAIT	fetomaternal alloimmune thrombocytopenia
FVW	flow velocity waveform
hCG	human chorionic gonadotrophin
IgG	immunoglobulin G
IgM	immunoglobulin M
IUGR	intrauterine growth restriction
MRI	magnetic resonance imaging
MoM	multiples of the median
Nd:YAG	neodymium:yttrium-aluminium-garnett
NIH	non-immune hydrops fetalis
NT	nuchal translucency
PAPP-A	pregnancy-associated plasma protein A
PCR	polymerase chain reaction
PI	pulsatility index
PKU	phenylketonuria
PO_2	partial pressure of oxygen
PPROM	preterm prelabour rupture of the membranes
Rh	rhesus
RI	resistance index
SGA	small for gestational age
SVT	supraventricular tachycardia
TRAP	twin reversed arterial perfusio
TTTS	twin-to-twin transfusion syndrome
uE_3	unconjugated oestriol

1 Screening for chromosomal abnormalities

Introduction

Screening for chromosomal abnormalities in an obstetric setting has traditionally meant screening for trisomy 21 (Down syndrome). Down syndrome has a live birth incidence of approximately 1:700 and is the single most common cause of mental restriction in school-age children. It is associated with a spectrum of mental and physical handicap and in view of this strategies have been developed to identify those pregnancies at 'high risk' of the condition. This affords the opportunity for subsequent diagnostic testing and termination of an affected pregnancy, if chosen by the parents. Screening for trisomy 21 is offered routinely as part of antenatal care and forms the major focus of discussion for this chapter.

The success of a screening programme is not measured only by the number of affected pregnancies detected. Screening for trisomy 21 should be performed on an 'opt-in' basis and parents should enter a screening programme only on the basis of adequate information about the implications and limitations of the test, so that they are not faced with results and decisions for which they are unprepared. Appropriate counselling is therefore essential to ensure that parents for whom screening is inappropriate do not enter the programme.

A screening test simply places the individual in a 'high-risk' or a 'low-risk' group. It does not tell us whether or not the condition being screened for is actually present. Therefore, a woman who has a 'high-risk' screening test result for trisomy 21 would have to undergo a diagnostic test if she wished to establish whether or not the pregnancy was affected. Similarly, a 'low-risk' result does not exclude the presence of trisomy 21; there is no such thing as 'no-risk' on the basis of a screening test result.

Development of screening programmes

Screening programmes have advanced from a single marker – maternal age – to using a combination of markers including biochemical and ultrasound features. In addition, there has been a drive to offer screening at earlier gestations. These aspects of screening programmes will be discussed in turn.

Table 1.1 The frequency of trisomy 21 at birth and at mid-trimester (time of amniocentesis) according to maternal age (Connor and Ferguson 1997)

Maternal age (years)	Frequency at birth	Frequency mid-trimester
20	1 in 1500	1 in 1200
25	1 in 1350	1 in 1000
30	1 in 900	1 in 700
35	1 in 380	1 in 300
37	1 in 240	1 in 200
39	1 in 150	1 in 120
41	1 in 85	1 in 70
45	1 in 28	1 in 22

MATERNAL AGE

Ninety-five percent of cases of trisomy 21 are due to non-disjunction, an abnormality of meiotic division, and the risk is known to increase with advancing maternal age. The risk of trisomy 21 increases relatively gradually up until the age of 35 years, after which time the increase in risk is much steeper (Table 1.1). The first screening programme for trisomy 21 was therefore based on maternal age, since it was estimated that approximately 30% of trisomy 21 pregnancies occurred to mothers ≥ 35 years old. However, since not all women in this age group opted for diagnostic testing (i.e. amniocentesis) actual detection rates were much lower than the potential 30%.

BIOCHEMICAL SCREENING

Second trimester

Alpha-fetoprotein (α-FP) was the first serum marker to be used in screening programmes for trisomy 21. α-FP is a fetal-specific protein that is produced initially by the fetal yolk sac and subsequently by the fetal liver. Biochemical screening has traditionally been performed between 15 and 21 weeks of gestation, during which time maternal serum levels of α-FP increase secondary to transport across the placenta and amnion. In pregnancies affected by trisomy 21, α-FP levels are reduced compared with unaffected pregnancies, and maternal serum α-FP in combination with age increased detection rates to approximately 40%.

In screening programmes, marker levels are described in multiples of the median (MOM) to allow for the fact that levels vary with gestational age. Values are calculated by dividing an individual's marker level by the

Table 1.2 Second-trimester serum markers, median multiples of the median (MOM) in pregnancies affected by trisomy 21 (reproduced with permission from Wald *et al.* 1997a)

Marker	MOM in trisomy 21
α-fetoprotein	0.75
Human chorionic gonadotrophin (hCG)	2.06
Free βhCG	2.20
Unconjugated oestradiol	0.72
Inhibin A	1.92

median level of that marker for the relevant gestation. The use of MOM values allows results from different laboratories to be interpreted in a common manner and facilitates adjustments for variables that influence marker levels. The performance of a particular screening test is defined by its detection rate for a given false-positive rate, the latter being the percentage of unaffected pregnancies categorised as 'high risk' by the screening test and thus potentially subject to diagnostic testing.

A number of other serum markers are recognised to be of value in second-trimester screening for trisomy 21. These are intact human chorionic gonadotrophin (hCG) or its free β-subunit (free βhCG), unconjugated oestriol (uE_3) and inhibin A. Table 1.2 illustrates the effect of trisomy 21 on serum marker levels (Wald *et al.* 1997a). Screening programmes now use maternal age and a combination of markers. The

Table 1.3 Screening performance of various marker combinations, for a 5% false positive rate, in the second trimester (adapted with permission from Wald *et al.* 1997a)

Screening programme	Sensitivity (%)	OAPR
Maternal age (36 years)	30	1:130
Age + α-FP	37	1:105
Age + α-FP + hCG (double test)	59	1:65
Age + α-FP + hCG + uE_3 (triple test)	69	1:55
Age + α-FP + hCG + inhibin A	68	1:55
Age + α-FP + hCG + uE_3 + inhibin A (quadruple test)	76	1:55

α-FP = α-fetoprotein; hCG = human chorionic gonadotrophin; OAPR = odds of pregnancy being affected if screening test positive; uE_3 = unconjugated oestradiol 'double test' combines age with α-FP and hCG and has detection rates of approximately 60% for a 5% false-positive rate. The 'triple test' adds uE3 to this combination. Opinion varies about the role of uE3 in screening, ranging from no additional benefit to an increase in sensitivity of up to 10% (Crossley *et al.* 1993; Wald *et al.*, 1997a). The addition of inhibin A to the double or triple screening protocol could increase detection rates by 5% to 10%. Table 1.3 summarises the sensitivity of various marker combinations.

Factors affecting second-trimester screening

Ultrasound assessment of gestational age results in improved performance of serum markers compared with gestation based on menstrual history. A number of variables influence marker levels (Table 1.4). Adjustments are routinely made for maternal weight in screening programmes. Serum marker levels are higher in twin pregnancies. Biochemical screening in multiple pregnancy is obviously fraught with problems such as inability to predict the affected fetus, technicalities of diagnostic testing and subsequent management if there is a discordant anomaly. For these reasons it is not applicable. Women who have had a screen-positive result in a previous pregnancy are more likely to have a positive result in subsequent pregnancies; the likelihood of this is dependent upon the woman's age.

FIRST TRIMESTER

The role of biochemical markers for screening in the first trimester has been evaluated. All of the markers that have been considered for use in the second trimester have been investigated but only free βhCG and pregnancy-associated plasma protein A (PAPP-A) are clearly discriminatory. In contrast to the second trimester, intact hCG is of no

---

Table 1.4   Variables affecting biochemical screening serum markers

Variable	Serum marker
Maternal weight	α-FP and hCG inversely proportional to weight
Insulin-dependent diabetes	uE_3 inhibin A reduced Total/free βhCG unchanged α-FP ?significant effect
Afro-Caribbean race	α-FP, hCG increased
Smoking	Total and free βhCG reduced α-FP increased

α-FP = α-fetoprotein; hCG = human chorionic gonadotrophin; uE_3 = unconjugated oestradiol

Table 1.5   First-trimester biochemical markers: median multiples of the median (MOM) in pregnancies affected by trisomy 21 (reproduced with permission from Wald *et al.* 1997a)

Marker	Median MOM
Free βhCG	1.83
PAPP-A	0.38

hCG = human chorionic gonadotrophin; PAPP-A = pregnancy-associated plasma protein A

value in first-trimester screening. In pregnancies affected by trisomy 21, free βhCG levels are increased and PAPP-A levels are reduced compared with unaffected pregnancies (Table 1.5). After 13 weeks of gestation, PAPP-A loses its discrimination as a screening marker. First-trimester serum screening programmes combining maternal age, free βhCG and PAPP-A with detection rates of 60–68% have been reported, using a risk cut-off level of 1:250, for a false positive rate of approximately 5% (Krantz *et al.* 1996; Wald *et al.* 1996).

ULTRASOUND SCREENING

Second trimester

The association between structural abnormalities and chromosome anomalies is well recognised. Approximately one-third of fetuses with trisomy 21 have major structural malformations (Table 1.6). Congenital heart defects are the most frequent anomaly (incidence 45%), atrioventricular canal and ventricular septal defects being most common. Employing cardiac anomaly as a screening marker would lead to significantly lower detection rates than current second-trimester biochemical screening programmes. In reality, only 33% of structural malformations in fetuses with trisomy 21 are detected antenatally, reducing the sensitivity of screening based on identification of structural anomaly even further. In view of this, attention has focused on the identification of 'soft markers' that might indicate an increased risk of trisomy 21.

Table 1.6 illustrates some of the 'soft markers' that have been identified ultrasonically in fetuses with trisomy 21. Soft markers are minor ultrasound findings, some of which are transient. Nuchal fold thickness is the most sensitive and specific second-trimester ultrasound marker, a measurement of ≥ 6 mm identifying approximately 40% of cases of trisomy 21 in a 'high-risk' population (Benacerraf 1996). The risk of aneuploidy increases with the number of anomalies detected, and multiple fetal anomalies may be associated with a risk of aneuploidy as

Table 1.6 Examples of ultrasound features associated with trisomy 21

Type of feature	Example
Structural	Cystic hygroma
	Atrioventricular septal defect
	Ventricular septal defect
	Duodenal atresia
	Ventriculomegaly
	Exomphalos
	Hydrothorax
Soft markers	Nuchal fold thickening
	Renal pyelectasis
	Short humerus
	Short femur
	Echogenic bowel
	Echogenic intracardiac focus
	Hypoplasia of middle phalanx fifth finger
	Sandal gap

high as 35% (Rizzo *et al*. 1990). It has been estimated that for a woman with a 'high-risk' biochemical screening result the risk of trisomy 21 is increased by approximately five-fold if a scan is also abnormal (Nyberg *et al*. 1995). However, a normal scan does not exclude a chromosomal problem since only 50% of fetuses with trisomy 21 had abnormal scan findings in this study.

The best combination of markers is nuchal fold thickness, short humerus and renal pyelectasis, which when present together have a sensitivity of 87% (false positive rate 6.7%) for detection of trisomy 21 (Vintzileos *et al*. 1997). The advantage of using these markers is that they are relatively easy to identify, in contrast with cardiac abnormalities, which require a more time-consuming scan and a greater level of expertise.

The most important point about the data available regarding ultrasound screening for chromosomal abnormalities is that it has been obtained from studies in 'high-risk' populations. The few prospective data that are available in 'low-risk' populations indicate that detection rates are certainly not as high. Large prospective studies are required to establish the role of second-trimester ultrasound screening in the general population.

First trimester

Nuchal translucency is the description given to the ultrasonic appearance of the fluid-filled space between the fetal skin and the soft tissue overlying the cervical spine (Figure 1.1). It is measured between 10 and 14 weeks

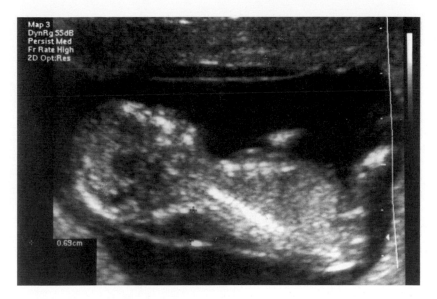

Figure 1.1 Increased nuchal translucency measurement

of gestation, optimally between 11 and 13 weeks. Prerequisites for nuchal translucency measurement are as follows (Snijders *et al.* 1998):

- crown–rump length 38–84 mm
- good sagittal view
- fetus occupies ≥ 75% of the image, neutral position
- ultrasound machine has 0.1-mm calipers
- maximum thickness of the subcutaneous translucency between the skin and soft tissue overlying the cervical spine is measured
- distinguish between fetal skin and amnion.

A number of studies have demonstrated an association between increased nuchal translucency thickness (Figure 1.2) and abnormal karyotype (Chitty and Pandya 1997). In the first trimester of normal pregnancy nuchal translucency thickness increases with advancing gestation. The 95th centile for nuchal translucency thickness is 0.8 mm above the normal median throughout the gestational range of 10–14 weeks. Therefore, it is the difference between the nuchal translucency measurement and the appropriate normal median for gestation that is incorporated into the model to calculate trisomy 21 risk. A large multicentre study of an unselected population has demonstrated that nuchal translucency measurement in combination with maternal age will identify a 'high-risk' group in which 77% of cases of trisomy 21 are detected for a 5% false positive rate (Snijders *et al.* 1998).

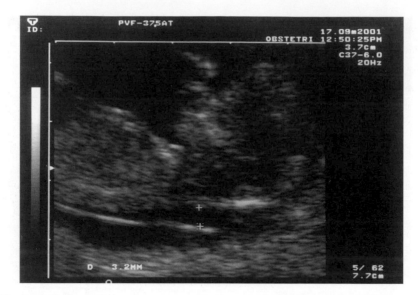

Figure 1.2 Nuchal translucency measurement, indicated by the calipers

Potential problems with nuchal translucency screening for trisomy 21 have been identified. It may be difficult to obtain a measurement if the fetal position is incorrect or there is maternal adiposity, in which case the scan will have to be prolonged or repeated. The effect of this on the management of ultrasound departments and antenatal clinics needs to be considered when introducing such a programme. Concerns have also been raised regarding the reproducibility of the measurement, highlighting the need for training and audit to ensure that the quality of screening programmes is equivalent between centres.

NUCHAL TRANSLUCENCY AND BIOCHEMICAL SCREENING

The latest advance in screening for trisomy 21 has been a combination of first-trimester nuchal translucency measurement and biochemical markers. In several studies the combination of free βhCG, PAPP-A, nuchal translucency and maternal age has been described with reported sensitivities of 80–89% for detection of trisomy 21 (Wald *et al.* 1997b; Spencer *et al.* 1999). These are substantially higher detection rates than second-trimester biochemical screening, for the same false positive rate. It has been calculated that the detection rate of a first-trimester programme should be 8.3% higher if it is to be considered superior to second-trimester screening (Dunstan *et al.* 1998), and the addition of nuchal translucency to first-trimester biochemistry clearly meets this criterion. First-trimester screening strategies are summarised in Table 1.7.

Table 1.7 Sensitivity of first-trimester screening programmes, for a 5% false positive rate

Screening programme	Sensitivity (%)
Maternal age + free βhCG	38
Age + PAPP-A	52
Age + PAPP-A + free βhCG	60
Age + nuchal translucency	77
Age + nuchal translucency + PAPP-A + free βhCG	89

hCG = human chorionic gonadotrophin; PAPP-A = pregnancy-associated plasma protein A; uE_3 = unconjugated oestradiol

First-trimester versus second-trimester screening

One of the main reasons for developing first-trimester screening options has been the perceived advantage that earlier detection of chromosomal abnormalities, and hence earlier termination of pregnancy by a surgical method, is less emotionally traumatic for the woman. Whether or not this is the case, and obviously different women will feel differently about this part of their care, certain aspects of first-trimester screening should be considered.

There is a natural attrition rate for aneuploid pregnancies as gestation advances and thus first-trimester screening will identify a proportion of pregnancies that were destined to miscarry spontaneously. This criticism obviously also applies to second-trimester programmes, but the rate of intrauterine lethality is higher between 12 weeks of gestation and term (31%) compared with 16 weeks and term (24%) (Morris *et al.* 1999). There is evidence to indicate that the intrauterine lethality in cases of trisomy 21 is higher in those fetuses with the biggest nuchal translucency measurements, demonstrating that this ultrasound marker will detect a number of pregnancies that would otherwise miscarry spontaneously. Therefore, the potential advantage of earlier termination of pregnancy has to be weighed against the fact that first-trimester screening will 'convert' a proportion of spontaneous miscarriages to pregnancy terminations, and the psychological impact of this factor needs to be considered.

Chorionic villus sampling (CVS) is the diagnostic procedure for karyotyping in the first trimester. It is technically more demanding than amniocentesis and, in general, a higher procedure-related loss rate is reported (1–2% versus 0.5–1.0%). Also, the rate of mosaicism is higher with CVS, necessitating a subsequent amniocentesis in a small proportion of pregnancies.

Women who have had a karyotypically abnormal pregnancy are

traditionally offered diagnostic testing in subsequent pregnancies. As discussed above, first-trimester screening will permit the identification of a number of aneuploid pregnancies that were destined to miscarry spontaneously, following which karyotyping would not be a routine issue in future pregnancies. Therefore, first-trimester screening will identify a group of women who will be faced with decisions regarding prenatal diagnostic testing in future pregnancies who would not have been identified by a second-trimester programme.

Screening for other chromosomal abnormalities

BIOCHEMISTRY

Currently, biochemical screening programmes for chromosomal abnormalities are aimed towards detection of trisomy 21, and women are counselled to this effect. However, it is recognised that other chromosomal anomalies are associated with altered marker levels compared with unaffected pregnancies. In trisomy 18, α-FP and hCG levels are both reduced and they can be used to calculate a specific risk for an individual pregnancy. Such screening protocols for trisomy 18, based on two or three marker combinations, have detection rates of 60% for a low false-positive rate (0.5%) (Hackshaw et al. 1995). While specific screening protocols are not available for other aneuploidies, trisomy 13 is associated with low α-FP levels and high hCG levels are associated with triploidy, and Turner syndrome (45XO) if hydrops is present.

ULTRASOUND

Increased nuchal translucency is a marker for other chromosomal abnormalities in addition to trisomy 21, including trisomies 18 and 13, 45XO, sex aneuploidies, triploidy, mosaicism and unbalanced translocations. A review of studies in unselected populations has estimated a mean detection rate for all aneuploidies of 70% (Chitty and Pandya 1997).

As indicated earlier, fetuses with chromosomal abnormalities frequently have significant structural malformations. It has been demonstrated that 100% of fetuses with trisomy 13 and 77% of fetuses with trisomy 18 have structural anomalies that may be amenable to detection by second-trimester ultrasound. However, in reality only 25% of aneuploid fetuses are detected by second-trimester structural survey in an unselected population (Chitty and Pandya 1997).

CONCLUSION

Significant developments have taken place in screening for trisomy 21 and various options are now available to couples in the antenatal period.

Each programme has its own advantages and disadvantages. Further advances are likely with expanding medical and scientific technology. Irrespective of future progress, the central issue to the success of any screening programme is appropriate counselling regarding the aims and limitations of the test so that couples can 'opt-in' to the programme on the basis of adequate information.

References

Benacerraf BR (1996) The second-trimester fetus with Down syndrome: detection using sonographic features. *Ultrasound Obstet Gynecol* **7**:147–55.

Chitty LS, Pandya PP. (1997) Ultrasound screening for fetal abnormalities in the first trimester. *Prenat Diagn* **17**:1269–81.

Connor M, Ferguson-Smith M, editors. (1997) *Essential Medical Genetics*. 5th ed. Oxford: Blackwell Science.

Crossley JA, Aitken DA, Connor JM. (1993) Second-trimester unconjugated oestriol levels in maternal serum from chromosomally abnormal pregnancies using an optimized assay. *Prenat Diagn* **13**:271–80.

Dunstan FDJ, Nix ABJ. (1998) Screening for Down's syndrome: the effect of test date on the detection rate. *Ann Clin Biochem* **35**:57–61.

Hackshaw AK, Kennard A, Wald NJ. (1995) Detection of pregnancies with trisomy 18 in screening programmes for Down's syndrome. *J Med Screen* **2**:228–9.

Krantz DA, Larsen JW, Buchanan PD, Macri JN. (1996) First-trimester Down syndrome screening: Free β-human chorionic gonadotrophin and pregnancy-associated plasma protein A. *Am J Obstet Gynecol* **174**:612–16.

Morris JK, Wald NJ, Watt HC. (1999) Fetal loss in Down syndrome pregnancies. *Prenat Diagn* **19**:142–5.

Nyberg DA, Luthy DA, Cheng EY, Sheley RC, Resta RG, Williams MA. (1995) Role of prenatal ultrasonography in women with positive screen for Down syndrome on the basis of maternal serum markers. *Am J Obstet Gynecol* **173**:1030–5.

Rizzo N, Pattalis MC, Pilu G, Orsini LF, Porolo A, Bovicelli L. (1990) Prenatal karyotype of malformed fetuses. *Prenat Diagn* **10**:17–23.

Snijders RJM, Noble P, Sebire N, Souka A, Nicolaides KH. (1998) UK multicentre project on assessment of risk of trisomy 21 by maternal age and fetal nuchal translucency thickness at 10–14 weeks gestation. *Lancet* **351**:343–6.

Spencer K, Souter V, Tul N, Snijders R, Nicolaides KH. (1999) A screening programme for trisomy 21 at 10–14 weeks using fetal nuchal translucency, maternal serum free β-human chorionic gonadotrophin and pregnancy associated plasma protein-A. *Ultrasound Obstet Gynecol* **13**:231–7.

Vintzileos AM, Campbell WA, Guzman ER, Smulian JC, McLean DA, Ananth CV. (1997) Second-trimester ultrasound markers for detection of trisomy 21: which markers are best? *Obstet Gynecol* **89**:941–4.

Wald NJ, George L, Smith D, Densem JW, Petterson K. (1996) Serum screening for Down's syndrome between 8 and 14 weeks of pregnancy. *Br J Obstet Gynaecol* **103**:407–12.

Wald NJ, Kennard A, Hackshaw A, McGuire A. (1997a) Antenatal screening for Down's syndrome. *J Med Screen* **4**:181–246.

Wald NJ, Hackshaw AK. (1997b) Combining ultrasound and biochemistry in first-trimester screening for Down's syndrome. *Prenat Diagn* **17**:821–9.

2 Prenatal diagnostic techniques

Introduction

Amniocentesis was first introduced into obstetric practice almost 50 years ago as a means of assessing the severity of rhesus (Rh) isoimmunisation by Bevis (1956). Since the 1970s, however, the severity of Rh disease has more commonly been investigated by cordocentesis, fetal blood sampling and the direct estimation of fetal haemoglobin, bilirubin and other parameters, with amniocentesis now being carried out most commonly in the middle trimester as a means of obtaining fetal cells for cytogenetic analysis.

CVS or biopsy was initially developed as an ultrasound-guided first-trimester diagnostic investigation using the transcervical route. More recently, the transabdominal route has been favoured and CVS now has an established place beside amniocentesis as a prenatal diagnostic technique. These invasive prenatal techniques are used as a means of obtaining fetal cells for cytogenetic analysis, amniocentesis being the technique of choice in the middle trimester, with optimum timing being between 15 and 16 weeks, and chorionic villus biopsy in the first trimester, ideally at 11–12 weeks.

Cordocentesis as a method of fetal blood sampling was first introduced using fetoscopic control in the 1960s but is now carried out using ultrasonic guidance. Although cordocentesis has to some extent been superseded by molecular biological techniques on fetal tissue obtained by less invasive means including amniocentesis and CVS, it still has a place in the investigation of some infective and haematological disorders.

Indications for prenatal diagnosis

Invasive prenatal diagnosis was introduced into clinical practice in the 1970s, primarily as a means of detecting trisomy 21 (Down syndrome). Maternal age, with a cut-off of 35 years being the most commonly adopted guideline, was the most commonly accepted indication at that time. A past history of chromosomal abnormality was also considered to be a valid indication. However, screening tests based on maternal biochemical parameters such as the triple test, which depends upon the measurement of maternal serum hCG, uE_3 and α-FP levels, have been widely adopted, together with screening by means of ultrasound nuchal translucency measurements. These screening tests and others are discussed in more detail in Chapter 1.

The use of these preliminary screening tests means that prenatal diagnosis can be offered to pregnant women of all ages. When maternal age alone was used as an indication, a relatively small number of trisomy 21 and other chromosomally abnormal pregnancies were diagnosed. This is because, although pregnancies in women over 35 years of age are more commonly affected by chromosomal abnormalities, such pregnancies are relatively uncommon, accounting for less than 10% of the total number. This percentage is, however, rising in developed countries, where there is quite a sharply rising mean maternal age.

Preliminary screening tests should be offered only after adequate counselling. Such counselling must include explanations as to the difference between screening and diagnostic investigations, as well as explanations relating to the limitations of screening and the implications of a 'positive' or 'negative' result.

The use of screening tests is discussed further in Chapter 1; for the purposes of this chapter, it should be noted that the cut-off for 'high' risk of a trisomy 21 pregnancy is most commonly set at one in 250, regardless of whether biochemical or ultrasonic screening is used.

It is crucially important that each patient and her partner are given a full explanation with regard to how the results of screening tests will be communicated to them and how they can seek further counselling, in particular if the screening test results show there to be a 'high' risk of abnormality and hence a necessity for the consideration of a diagnostic test. The services of a prenatal diagnosis coordinator and trained counsellors are invaluable in this context.

A large amount of information is given to the patient and her partner at the consultation stage. As this includes a quantity of possibly indigestible statistics, some of which may be initially difficult to understand, explanatory booklets for the various screening and diagnostic tests should also be provided.

The invasive diagnostic investigations carry a procedure-related fetal loss rate and correctly phrased written consent must be obtained for the specific procedure being used. As with screening tests, clear explanations must be provided with regard to the way in which results are to be communicated to the patient, and contact numbers provided so that the help of counselling services can be rapidly and reliably sought if necessary.

Amniocentesis

Amniocentesis has become established as the mid-trimester diagnostic investigation of choice since the mid-1970s. When amniocentesis was first introduced into clinical practice for the investigation of Rh isoimmunisation and later for the short-lived technique of estimating the lecithin–sphingomyelin ratio as a means of estimating lung maturity, a 'blind' technique without ultrasonic control was commonly used. Mid-trimester amniocentesis as used today for diagnostic purposes must be carried out under ultrasonic control so that the tip of the operator's needle is visible all the time (Figure 2.1) (RCOG 2000). This should ensure that damage to the fetus is prevented. A 22-gauge spinal needle is usually the instrument of choice. Local anaesthesia is not necessary.

The operator should try to avoid the placenta but it is more important to gain access to a deep, clear pool of liquor, even if this does mean a transplacental approach, than to go for a more inaccessible pool clear of the placenta and risk either a failed tap or the need for a second puncture, which has been shown to increase the risk of post-amniocentesis miscarriage. If a transplacental tap is necessary, the cord insertion must be avoided (RCOG 2000). Mid-trimester amniocentesis is normally carried out between 15 and 17 weeks of gestational age, the gestational age having been determined ultrasonically as well as by means of menstrual

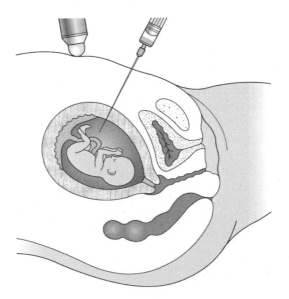

Figure 2.1 Amniocentesis

dating. Fetal viability will have been checked prior to insertion of the spinal needle and the skin cleansed with antiseptic fluid.

Patients understandably find amniocentesis a nerve-racking procedure and appreciate being 'talked through' the technique, with warning as to when the needle is going to be inserted. They will almost invariably appreciate a companion to provide moral support. Following withdrawal of the stilette, 15–17 ml of amniotic fluid are withdrawn and the needle is swiftly removed. Great care must be taken in labelling the specimen. The patient's blood group must be checked, as she will need an injection of anti-D immunoglobulin 250 iu if she is Rh-negative to prevent Rh isoimmunisation, and she will be warned to be on the lookout for blood or liquor loss vaginally, vaginal bleeding and unexpected pain or fever. If any of these circumstances obtain, she should be asked to contact appropriate medical help – in most cases this will be the delivery unit of the hospital concerned.

Cytogenetic analysis

The techniques for cytogenetic analysis are beyond the scope of this chapter – suffice it to say that culture of the cells that are separated from the supernatant fluid by centrifugation will normally be successful in 98–99% of cases. Recent technological advances have allowed the rapid analysis of uncultured amniotic fluid cells by fluorescence *in situ* hybridisation (FISH). By this means, trisomy 13, 18, 21 and sex-chromosome abnormalities have been detected, with results available within 24 hours of the specimen being received (Eiben *et al.* 1999).

RISKS

The major hazard of amniocentesis is pregnancy loss. The results of the largest randomised single-centre study of amniocentesis were published in 1986 (Tabor *et al.* 1986). This study involved over 4600 women who were below the cut-off age at which amniocentesis was normally offered at that time and hence regarded as low risk. They were randomised into 'non-amniocentesis' and 'amniocentesis' groups; a standard technique using an 18-gauge needle with ultrasonic guidance was used and the procedure was carried out at 16–18 weeks. The amniocentesis group had a procedure-related fetal loss rate that was 1% higher than the loss rate in the non-amniocentesis group. As this is the only randomised trial of the procedure ever carried out, and as such a trial is unlikely to be ever repeated, this figure is widely quoted in counselling patients (Tabor *et al.* 1986). There is no evidence that amniocentesis carried out between 16 and 18 weeks is associated with a significant risk of orthopaedic problems such as talipes or with intrauterine infection.

TIMING

The use of early amniocentesis (prior to 14 weeks) has been reviewed by Wilson (2000) and Alfirevic (2000a). These major review articles included studies of trials including the Canadian Early and Mid-trimester Amniocentesis Trial (CEMAT 1998), in which women were randomly allocated to early (11–12 weeks plus six days) or mid-trimester (15–16 weeks plus six days). In this large prospective randomised trial several areas of concern were identified, including an increased fetal loss rate for early as opposed to mid-trimester amniocentesis (7.6% as opposed to 5.9% total fetal loss rates), an increase in talipes in the early amniocentesis group (1.3% as opposed to 0.1%) and an increased incidence of amniotic fluid leakage (3.5% as opposed to 1.7%). There was also a greater number of culture failures in the early amniocentesis group and these procedures were generally judged to be more difficult – but not as technically demanding as transabdominal CVS. Nevertheless, in the review (Alfirevic 2000a) comparing early amniocentesis and transabdominal CVS based on three randomised control trials carried out by Alfirevic, each of which showed an increased miscarriage and talipes rate, the reviewer concluded that at the present time it would seem prudent to offer amniocentesis as the routine method for prenatal diagnosis after 14 weeks and to offer CVS as the routine method of invasive prenatal diagnostic investigation between 11 and 13 weeks (Alfirevic 2000a).

Chorionic villus sampling

This technique was first described as a means of first-trimester sex-chromosome determination in China (Tietung Hospital 1975). The technique was first introduced into the West by a team at St Mary's Hospital in London (Horwell *et al.* 1983) and has subsequently been developed, in particular by Brambati and his team in Italy (Firth *et al.* 1991). Worldwide data are analysed in the International CVS Registry, which had accumulated details of 130 000 CVS cases from more than 180 centres by the end of 1996. The World Health Organization regional office for Europe report concluded in 1992 that, in expert hands, CVS should be regarded as a safe, routine procedure. In 1991, however, there was concern following the publication of a small early first-trimester series in which limb-reduction defect cases were seen following CVS carried out prior to ten weeks (Brambati *et al.* 1987). The limb defects could be related to placental damage or embolisation and, although a WHO statement following an analysis of 80 000 cases carried out from eight completed weeks onwards failed to confirm the earlier findings, the original report, as well as two other reports (Burton *et al.* 1992; Brambati *et al.* 1992) showing clusters of limb defect cases, understandably caused a lot of anxiety and CVS is now carried out at 10–12 weeks rather than earlier.

TIMING

The generally accepted optimum gestational age for CVS is between 10 and 12 weeks. The placenta at this stage of pregnancy is easy to identify and of such thickness that safe sampling is usually possible. Although CVS can be carried out at later stages of pregnancy, second-trimester amniocentesis is generally preferred, because the technique is technically more straightforward, the pregnancy loss rate is generally held to be lower and because amniocentesis does not incur as high a risk of mosaicism.

TECHNIQUES

Most of the early trials of CVS relied on transcervical sampling but the transabdominal route has now become the technique of choice. This route is preferred by patients, has a lower rate of immediate complications such as vaginal bleeding, a lower risk of intrauterine infection and a shorter learning curve. There may, however, still be a case for the transcervical route, particularly if access to a low-lying posterior placenta is needed. Both forceps and cannulae have been used for transcervical aspiration and

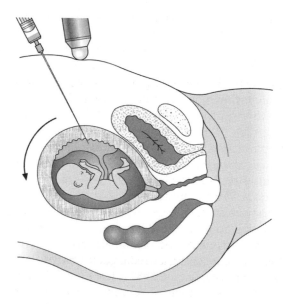

Figure 2.2 Chorionic villus biopsy in which needle is intentionally inserted into placenta

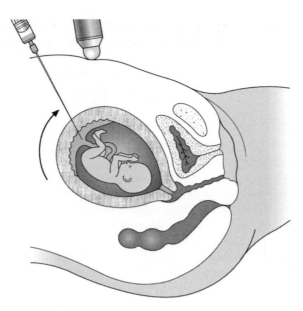

Figure 2.3 Chorionic villus biopsy

appear to provide comparable samples. There is not enough evidence to support a change to forceps for clinicians who have become familiar with the use of cannulae (Alfirevic 2000b).

Transabdominal CVS is most commonly carried out using a single 18–20-gauge spinal needle with a stilette inserted under continuous ultrasound control using a freehand ultrasound-guided approach. Following the use of lignocaine 1% local anaesthetic to infiltrate the abdominal wall, the needle is progressively inserted through the layers of the abdominal wall and the myometrium until the placenta is entered. It is then moved up and down five to ten times in the placental tissue with suction being applied via the aspirating syringe, which, together with the needle, should be partially filled with sterile saline to aid aspiration of villous material. Either a single-operator technique, with the operator holding the ultrasound transducer in one hand and the needle in the other, or a two-operator technique with a sonographer manipulating the transducer can be opted for; there is no evidence to suggest that either technique is superior.

An alternative technique using a needle guide attached to the ultrasound probe has also been described (Smidt-Jensen and Hahnemann 1988). Following aspiration, the needle is removed while still attached to the syringe and the sample injected into a culture medium for evaluation by the cytogeneticist, who should be waiting to perform immediate microscopy to assess the adequacy of the sample.

Access to an anterior placenta may be facilitated by a full bladder, which will usually push the uterus into an axial or slightly retroverted position (Figure 2.2). Sampling a posterior placenta will generally be helped by asking the patient to empty her bladder, which is usually followed by the uterus adopting a more anteverted position (Figure 2.3).

CONTRAINDICATIONS

Transabdominal CVS may be impossible to carry out if there are obstacles to the safe passage of the sampling needle, such as bowel attached to the abdominal wall or multiple fibroids. Transcervical CVS should not be carried out in the presence of vaginal or cervical infection. With either route it is wise to postpone the investigation if there is active bleeding suggestive of a possible threatened miscarriage. In Rh-negative patients anti-D immunoglobulin 250 iu must be administered following the procedure (RCOG 1999).

If technical difficulties are anticipated following scanning – for example, due to an inaccessible posterior placenta – or if the sample aspirated is deemed 'inadequate' by the cytogeneticist, it is preferable to defer further attempts at sampling for a week rather than persist with further attempts that may well be fruitless and increase the risk of miscarriage (Regan *et al.* 1993).

AMNIOCENTESIS OR CVS?

The advantages of first-trimester CVS as opposed to mid-trimester amniocentesis are obvious to most patients: the investigation can be carried out at an earlier stage of pregnancy, the results are equally accurate, and should termination be necessary, it may be possible for this to be carried out vaginally as a first-trimester procedure. Chorionic villi are also suitable for investigations other than cytogenetic analyses: the tissue is metabolically active and can thus be used in the diagnosis of many inherited metabolic diseases. The amount of DNA obtained from a conventional sample allows for many analyses using recombinant DNA technology and such analyses are not usually possible with amniotic fluid cells. CVS is, however, most commonly carried out at the present time as a sequel to first-trimester screening by means of nuchal translucency measurements combined with blood tests such as the beta subunit of hCG and PAPP-A – these techniques are described in greater detail in Chapter 1.

CVS may also be offered as a primary diagnostic technique for women in the older age group. No specific cut-off is recommended but some women, for example those over the age of 40 years, who have a high chance of a 'high-risk' screening test result because of their age, may decide to proceed directly to a diagnostic test rather than opt for the uncertainty and extra time involved in going through the screening process first.

RISKS

CVS has become an established diagnostic investigation technique with acceptable fetal loss rates that have been shown in most large trials to be no higher in terms of procedure-related loss than the losses associated with mid-trimester amniocentesis (Brambati *et al.* 1987; Regan *et al.* 1993). There is no evidence of an increased risk of congenital malformations when CVS is performed after the tenth completed week of pregnancy. Mid-trimester amniocentesis does, however, carry a lower procedure-related fetal loss rate, is easier to perform and possibly less painful. There are fewer problems with mosaicism but the diagnosis will not usually be available until 18 weeks or later.

CYTOGENIC ANALYSIS USING CHORIONIC VILLI

Immediate assessment by microscopy carried out by a cytogeneticist in the ultrasound/fetal medicine department is extremely advantageous in assessing the adequacy of the sample obtained at CVS and this cooperative approach is to be strongly advised. The sample will then either be cultured, a process that normally takes 10–15 days and is thereafter followed by chromosome banding techniques or subjected to rapid karyotyping, which may be performed by examining cytotrophoblastic cells arrested in metaphase either immediately after sampling or after short-term (24–48 hour) culture. Placental mosaicism may cause diagnostic dilemmas and the necessity for a second diagnostic procedure, but this eventuality is fortunately rare.

Invasive diagnostic techniques in multiple pregnancy

First-trimester CVS may be technically a more suitable procedure than mid-trimester amniocentesis as a means of obtaining fetal tissue for chromosomal analysis in twin or higher-order multiple pregnancies. This is because the membranes can be clearly identified at around 11–12 weeks. Dichorionic pregnancy can be diagnosed if two distinct placental sites are seen or, should the placenta be confluent, there is seen to be a membranous septal thickness of 2 mm or more. It is usually possible to obtain samples from both placentas under these circumstances but if technical problems arise in such cases referral to a fetal medicine centre should be seriously considered.

The relative risks of first-trimester CVS and mid-trimester amniocentesis in carrying out diagnostic procedures to obtain tissue for cytogenetic analysis have been compared. In cases with chromosomally normal fetuses and placentas, the total fetal loss rate was lower in the CVS series (Wapner *et al.* 1993). Amniocentesis may, however, be preferred by some operators and will not usually pose difficulties unless the membrane between the sacs is not clearly seen. If there is an extensive anterior placenta, transplacental needling may be necessary. This has not been shown to increase the risk of miscarriage in singleton pregnancies but could, in theory, increase the risk of miscarriage in multiple pregnancy, especially if a double-tap technique is necessary to aspirate fluid from each sac.

Cordocentesis

Cordocentesis as a method of fetal blood sampling was first carried out in the 1960s under fetoscopic guidance and carried a procedure-related fetal loss rate of over 5%. The first percutaneous umbilical cord sampling under ultrasound control was reported by Daffos *et al.* in 1983, and this development revolutionised the technique, allowing access to the fetal vascular compartment for both diagnostic and therapeutic means, with a procedure-related fetal loss rate comparable to other invasive prenatal diagnostic procedures. The place of fetal blood sampling has, however, diminished with advances in molecular biology, including the use of the polymerase chain reaction to obtain DNA samples obtained from fetal tissue obtained by less invasive techniques. Nevertheless, cord blood sampling still has a place in the investigation of fetal infection and the anaemia that can follow infections such as parvovirus, congenital toxoplasmosis (Naides and Weiner 1989) and Rh isoimmunisation. In Rh and also erythrocyte alloimmunisation, fetal blood sampling is the main tool used for diagnosis, estimating prognosis and providing treatment (Nicolaides *et al.* 1986). In cases of severe anaemia *in utero*, transfusion by means of cordocentesis using specially prepared red-cell concentrates is the treatment of choice. This is discussed in detail in Chapter 5.

Cordocentesis has been used to obtain a fetal blood sample as a means of obtaining a sample for rapid karyotyping in cases of mosaicism in chorionic villus or, more rarely, amniotic cell culture, or in some cases of ultrasonically diagnosed fetal abnormality. Rapid karyotyping by this means has now been partly superseded by rapid diagnostic procedures carried out on chorionic villi and amniocytes using molecular biological technology.

TECHNIQUES AND COMPLICATIONS

The umbilical vein is identified ultrasonically and either a biopsy guide or a freehand technique using a 20-gauge spinal needle under direct ultrasound control used (Figure 2.4). The procedure is technically more difficult and the loss rate higher if the procedure is carried out prior to 20 weeks (Weiner and Okamura 1996). Apart from the freehand technique, the use of a needle guide has been described (Weiner and Okamura 1996). The site of

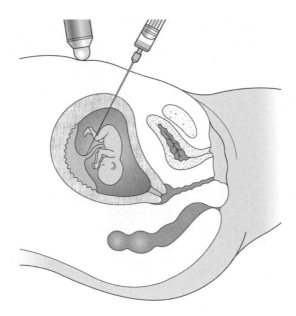

Figure 2.4 Cordocentesis in which needle is inserted into the umbilical vein where the umbilical cord goes into the placenta

cord insertion at the placenta, where the cord is relatively fixed, is the most favoured target for cordocentesis. Local anaesthesia is not generally used.

The major complication of cordocentesis is fetal bradycardia or occasionally asystole. The world experience of cordocentesis is of course much smaller than for other invasive techniques such as CVS or amniocentesis, but there are some large studies including that of Weiner and Okamura (1996), who studied the results of 1260 diagnostic cordocentesis performed at a mean gestational age of 29 weeks. The umbilical vein was successfully punctured in 90% of cases and there were 12 procedure-related losses (0.95%). This series involved the use of a needle guide; reported series using freehand techniques have shown similar or slightly higher fetal loss rates (Donner *et al.* 1994).

Fetal blood sampling still has a place in the investigation of some infective and anaemic syndromes and in experienced hands there is an acceptable fetal loss rate.

Audit of invasive prenatal diagnostic procedures

It is absolutely vital that units undertaking prenatal diagnostic procedures carry out regular accurate audits of their results to ascertain the success and complication rates of the various procedures carried out. Examples of

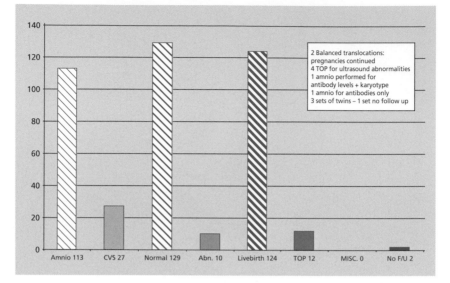

Figure 2.5 Prenatal diagnosis outcomes 1999: operator 1; Abn = abortion; Amnio = amniocentesis; CVS = chrionic villus sampling; F/U = follow up; TOP = termination of pregnancy

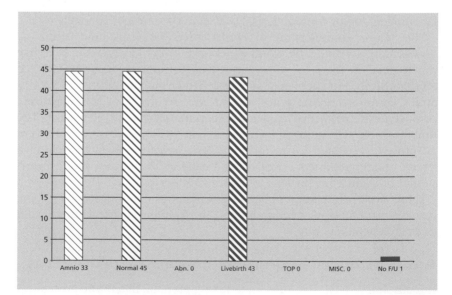

Figure 2.6 Prenatal diagnosis outcomes 1999: operator 2; Abn = abortion; Amnio = amniocentesis; F/U = follow up; TOP = termination of pregnancy

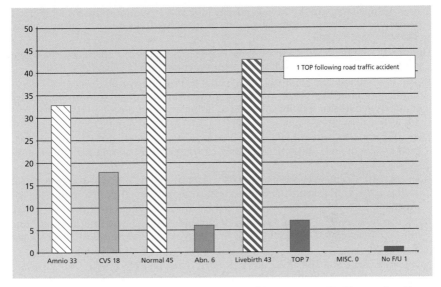

Figure 2.7 Prenatal diagnosis outcomes 1999: operator 3; Abn = abortion; Amnio = amniocentesis; CVS = chrionic villus sampling; F/U = follow up; TOP = termination of pregnancy

such audits are shown in Figures 2.5, 2.6 and 2.7 (Rosie Maternity Unit, Addenbrooke's, Cambridge, unpublished data), in which the results obtained in amniocentesis and CVS for three different operators were assessed over a calendar year. The use of such audits is essential if accurate evaluation of the service provided is to be obtained.

References

Alfirevic Z. (2000a) Early amniocentesis versus transabdominal chorion villus sampling for prenatal diagnosis. *Cochrane Database Syst Rev 2000*;(**3**):CD000077.

Alfirevic Z. (2000b) Instruments for transcervical chorionic villus sampling for prenatal diagnosis. *Cochrane Database Syst Rev 2000*;(**1**):CD000114.

Bevis DC. (1956) Blood pigments in haemolytic disease of the newborn. *J Obstet Gynaecol Br Emp* **63**:68–75.

Brambati B, Oldrini A, Ferrazzi E, Lanzani A. (1987) Chorionic villus sampling: an analysis of the obstetric experience of 1,000 cases. *Prenat Diagn* **7**:157–69.

Brambati, B., Simoni, G., Travi, M, Danesino C, Tului L, Privitera O. (1992) Genetic diagnosis by chorionic villus sampling before 8 gestational weeks: efficiency, reliability, and risks on 317 completed pregnancies. *Prenat Diagn* **12**, 789–99.

Burton BK, Schultz CJ, Burd LI. (1992) Limb anomalies associated with chorionic villus sampling. *Obstet Gynecol* **79**:726–30.

The Canadian Early and Mid-Trimester Amniocentesis Trial (CEMAT) Group. (1998) Randomised trial to assess safety and fetal outcome of early and midtrimester amniocentesis. *Lancet* **351**:242–7.

Daffos F, Capella-Pavlovsky M, Forestier F. (1983) A new procedure for fetal blood sampling *in utero*: preliminary results of fifty-three cases. *Am J Obstet Gynecol* **146**:985–7.

Donner, C., Simon, P., Karioun, A, Aviri F, Rodesch F. (1994) Experience of a single team of operators in 891 diagnostic funipunctures. *Obstet Gynecol* **84**, 827–31.

Eiben, B., Trawicki, W., Hammans W, Goebel R, Pruggmayer M, Epplen JT. (1999) Rapid prenatal diagnosis of aneuploidies in uncultured amniocytes by fluorescence in situ hybridization. Evaluation of > 3000 cases. *Fetal Diagn Ther* **14**, 193–7.

Firth HV, Boyd PA, Chamberlain P, MacKenzie IZ, Lindenbaum RH, Huson SM. (1991) Severe limb abnormalities after chorionic villus sampling at 56–66 days of gestation. *Lancet* **337**:762–3.

Horwell DH, Loeffler FE, Coleman DV. (1983) Assessment of a transcervical aspiration technique for chorionic villus biopsy in the first trimester of pregnancy. *Br J Obstet Gynaecol* **90**:196–8.

Naides SJ, Weiner CP. (1989) Antenatal diagnosis and palliative treatment of non-immune hydrops fetalis secondary to fetal parvovirus B19 infection. *Prenat Diagn* **9**:105–14.

Nicolaides KH, Soothill PW, Rodeck CH, Clewell W. (1986) Rh disease: intravascular fetal blood transfusion by cordocentesis. *Fetal Ther* **1**:185–92.

Regan L, Milton PJD, Waters J, Ferguson-Smith ME. (1993) Transabdominal chorionic villus sampling. In Macek M, Ferguson MA, Špála M, editors. *Early Fetal Diagnosis: Recent Progress and Public Health Implications*. Prague: Karolinum-Charles University Press; 1992. p. 123–4.

Royal College of Obstetricians and Gynaecologists. (2000) *Amniocentesis*. Guideline No. 8. London: RCOG; 2000.

Royal College of Obstetricians and Gynaecologists. (1999) *Use of Anti-D Immunoglobulin for Rh Prophylaxis*. Guideline No. 22. London: RCOG; 1999.

Smidt-Jensen S, Hahnemann N. (1988) Transabdominal sampling for fetal genetic diagnosis. Technical and obstetrical evaluation of 100 cases. *Prenat Diagn* **8**:7–17.

Tabor A, Philip J, Madsen M, Bang J, Obel EB, Norgaard-Pedersen B. (1986) Randomised controlled trial of genetic amniocentesis in 4606 low-risk women. *Lancet* **i**:1287–93.

Tietung Hospital of Ansham Iron and Steel Company (1975) Fetal sex prediction by sex chromatin of chorionic villi cells during early pregnancy. *Chinese Med J* **2**:118–25.

Wapner RJ, Johnson A, Davis G, Urban A, Morgan P, Jackson L. (1993) Prenatal diagnosis in twin gestations, a comparison between second-trimester amniocentesis and first-trimester chorionic villus sampling. *Obstet Gynecol* **82**:49–56.

Weiner CP, Okamura K. (1996) Diagnostic fetal blood sampling - technique-related losses. *Fetal Diagn Ther* **11**:169–75.

Wilson RD. (2000) Amniocentesis and chorionic villus sampling. *Curr Opin Obstet Gynecol 2000*:**12**:81–6.

3 The routine anomaly scan

Introduction

Approximately 2% of all births are affected by a fetal abnormality. In addition, 15–20% of perinatal deaths and deaths in the first year of life are a direct consequence of fetal abnormalities or their sequelae. For most parents fully expecting a 'normal' baby, this can prove difficult. Although it is well recognised that some women are at increased risk of a fetal abnormality (Table 3.1), over 90% of fetal abnormalities are found in 'low-risk women'. In view of this, many units have introduced a routine

Table 3.1   Maternal risk factors for congenital fetal abnormality

Maternal risk factors	Associated abnormalities
Retinoic acid therapy	Central nervous system Cardiovascular abnormalities Craniofacial defects Mental restriction
Anticonvulsant therapy	Central nervous system hydantoin syndrome Microcephaly
Anticoagulant therapy (warfarin)	Bone stippling Microcephaly
Maternal phenylketonuria	Neural tube defects Cardiovascular abnormalities Microcephaly
Maternal diabetes	Neural tube defects Cardiovascular abnormalities Sacral agenesis
Parental congenital heart disease	Cardiovascular abnormalities
Parental spina bifida (? lithium)	Neural tube defects Ebstein's abnormality Hydrocephalus Polyhydramnios

Table 3.2 Checklist for a second trimester routine anomaly scan

Structures examined	Features to be indentified
Head and neck	Complete cranial bones Thalamus and septum pellucidum Cerebellum: 2 lobes and vermis Thalamus and septum pellucidum Lateral ventricles: anterior and posterior horns Normal hemisphere ratios Choroid plexus Nuchal oedema and cisterna magna
Spine	Complete vertebrae seen in both transverse and coronal planes
Face	Normal facial profile Two orbits Lips and nostrils[a]
Chest	Position/size of heart Correct number/size of chambers Two atrioventricular valves
Abdomen	Stomach bubble on left of abdomen Unbilical cord root insertion Three vessels in cord[a] Integrity of diaphragm Kidneys: measure renal pelvis diameter Bladder
Limbs	Upper limbs x 2 Hands x 2 (5 digits each hand) Lower limbs x 2 Feet x 2 (5 digits each foot)

[a] denotes features that may not be examined in every unit

anomaly scan with a view to improving the detection rate of major abnormalities. Currently, around 80% of obstetric units in England and Wales offer this service (RCOG 1997).

Second-trimester anomaly scans

Second-trimester anomaly scans should be performed between 18 and 20 weeks of gestation. The main features that should be examined are listed in Table 3.2 and illustrated in Figures 3.1 (a–j). On many occasions even these specific features may be difficult to visualise, most commonly due to

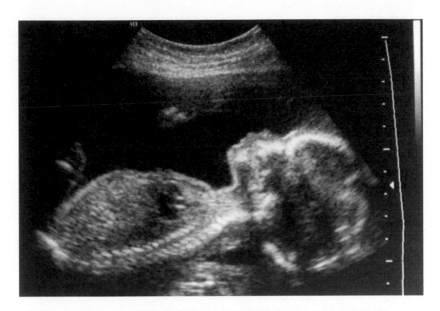

Figure 3.1(a) A longitudinal section through the fetus at 18 weeks of gestation demonstrating a normal facial profile

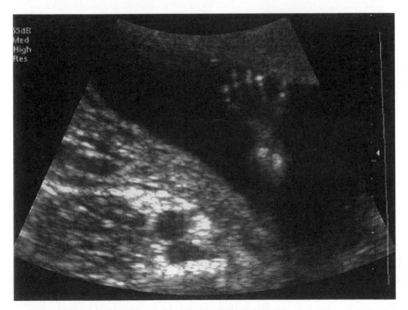

Fig 3.1(b) An open fetal hand with five fingers

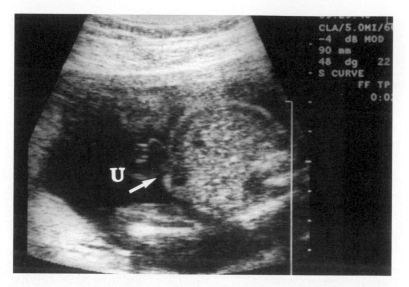

Fig 3.1(c) A transverse section of the fetal abdomen; the umbilical cord (U) is seen to enter the fetal abdomen directly and the surrounding skin is complete

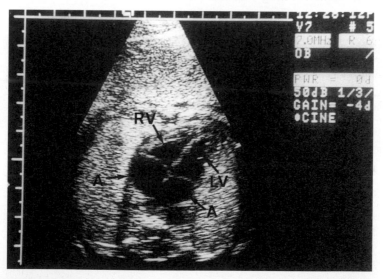

Fig 3.1(d) A transverse section of the fetal chest at 18 weeks gestation; the fetal heart points to the left and occupies less than one-third of the chest; the right ventricle (RV) sits under the anterior chest wall and is of similar size to the left ventricle (LV); both atria are equal in size; the tricuspid valve (TV) is inserted nearer the apex of the heart and the mitral valve (MV) giving an offset appearance at the crux of the heart

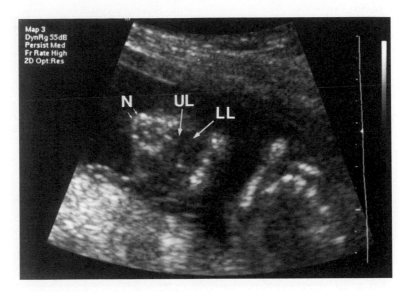

Fig 3.1(e) A frontal image of the fetal face illustrating the fetal nose (N), upper lip (UL) and lower lip (LL)

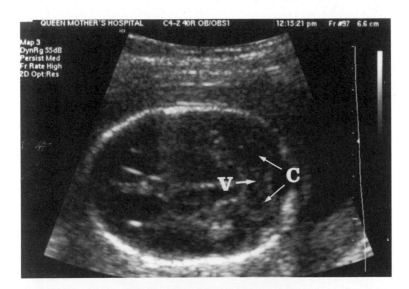

Fig 3.1(f) A transverse section of a normal oval-shaped fetal head demonstrating the two lobes of cerebellum (C) connected by the vermis (V); the posterior horn of the lateral ventricle is also outlined (P) and measures less than half the diameter of the hemisphere

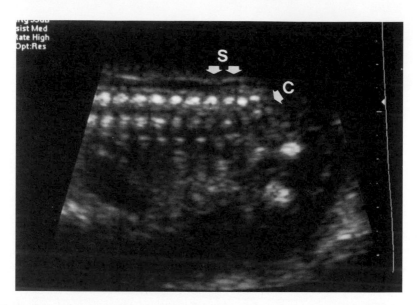

Fig 3.1(g) The fetal spine in longitudinal section with the two vertebral columns merging together at the fetal coccyx (C); a complete layer of skin (S) is seen to overlie the vertebral bones

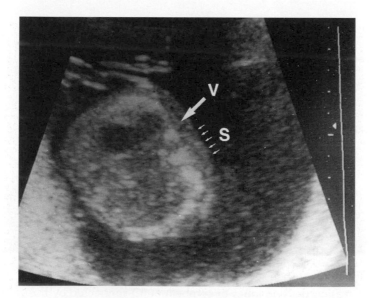

Fig 3.1(h) A transverse section of the fetal spine illustrating the three points of the vertebral bones (V) and an intact skin layer (S)

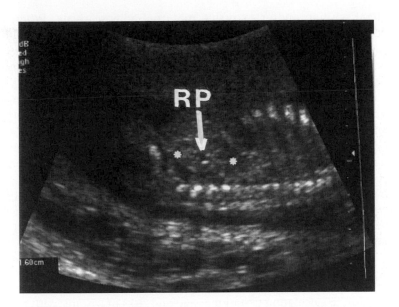

Fig 3.1(i) A longitudinal section through a normal fetal kidney; the renal pelvis (RP) is central and the surrounding renal tissue has a lobular appearance

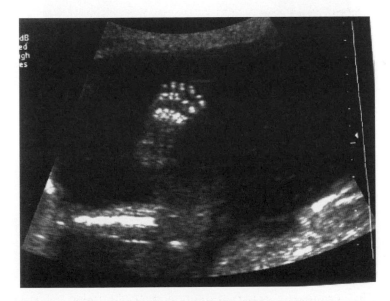

Fig 3.1(j) The sole of the fetal foot with five toes identified

the fetal position and/or excessive maternal adipose tissue. When the anatomical survey is not complete at one visit, further scans should be arranged. Although detailed scans performed prior to 18 weeks of gestation permit an early diagnosis of problems, they are time-consuming and are more likely to be incomplete.

While there appears to be a great diversity in the anomaly detection rate reported by different groups, most units identify 50–70% of severe or lethal anomalies antenatally (Chitty *et al.* 1991; Luck 1992; Boyd *et al.* 1998). It is clear that appropriate training in detailed ultrasound scanning and specific training in cardiac imaging does improve the antenatal detection rate achieved (Sharland *et al.* 1992; Shirley 1992). Despite this and the continual improvements in image resolution, some cases of congenital heart disease, diaphragmatic hernia, skeletal dysplasias and other anomalies will always remain undetected, since many will not manifest themselves until the third trimester or postnatal life.

The first-trimester anomaly scan

In addition to calculating gestational age and risks of trisomy with nuchal translucency, some studies (e.g. Braithwaite *et al.* 1996) have also used

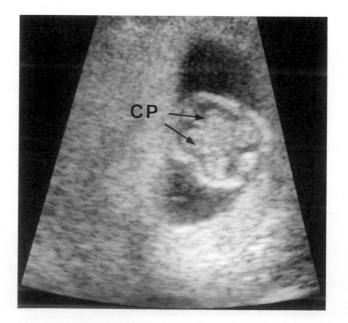

Fig 3.2 The first-trimester fetal brain; the choroid plexus (CP) completely fills the lateral ventricles, which occupy most of cranial hemisphere

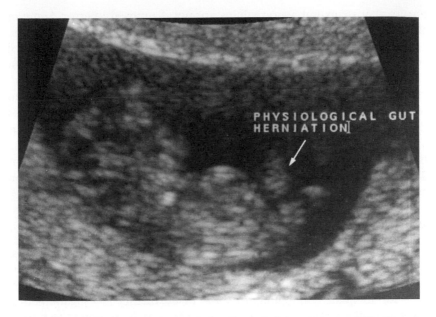

Figure 3.3 A transverse section of the fetal abdomen; the umbilical cord (U) is seen to enter the fetal abdomen directly and the surrounding skin is complete

the first trimester (11–14 weeks of gestation) examination for the detection of structural abnormalities. An anatomical examination, as described in Table 3.2, is completed initially with a transabdominal ultrasound scan. In 20–30% of cases, the views obtained will be unsatisfactory and transvaginal ultrasound will also be required to complete the anatomical survey. The ultrasound appearances of the intracranial anatomy, central nervous system and gastrointestinal tract are quite different from those seen in the second trimester. In particular, within the cranium, the choroid plexus is relatively large and occupies most of the lateral ventricle, which in turn occupies most of the hemisphere. This appearance does not indicate hydrocephalus. In addition, the fetal intra-abdominal contents will normally herniate into the amniotic cavity until around 11 weeks of gestation. At times, the return to the abdominal cavity may be delayed or the bowel may appear to herniate into the base of the cord root. Once again, these may be 'normal' features and do not necessarily indicate an anterior abdominal wall defect unless the appearances persist once the fetal crown–rump length is greater than 68 mm. Those performing first-trimester detailed scans must appreciate these normal embryological developments to ensure that structural abnormalities are not diagnosed in error. Some of these are illustrated in Figures 3.2 and 3.3.

A detailed scan in the first trimester using the regimen described above will detect 50–60% of structural abnormalities (Whitlow *et al.* 1999). Cranial, neck and gastrointestinal abnormalities are reliably identified, while spina bifida, cardiac and skeletal problems are more difficult to recognise. It should be noted that many of these anomalies are also difficult to detect in the second trimester. The use of transvaginal scans as a first-line approach in the first trimester does not appear to improve the detection rates achieved, since there is a limited range of movement available with the probe and adequate examination depends largely on appropriate fetal orientation and movement at the time of scanning.

Aims of routine anomaly scans

For the majority of parents, a routine anomaly scan will exclude most major structural anomalies and reassure them regarding their pregnancy. In those pregnancies where a problem is identified, early diagnosis offers time for adequate counselling. In some cases, further investigations or a second opinion from a fetal medicine centre may be indicated to ensure that the prospective parents have accurate information on the likely outcome for their pregnancy. When lethal or severe abnormalities are identified, many parents will not wish to continue with the pregnancy and the process of termination of pregnancy should be discussed.

Other parents will wish to continue with a pregnancy irrespective of the severity of the problem seen. Once again, an early diagnosis can give parents time to prepare for events after delivery and it gives clinicians the opportunity to plan the timing and the most appropriate place for delivery.

For the future, fetal surgery for conditions such as diaphragmatic hernia depends on an early antenatal diagnosis. With improved operator experience and increasing use of routine anomaly scanning in both the first and second trimester it is hoped that fetal therapy and surgery will become a real option for certain conditions in the next few years.

Problems associated with routine anomaly scans

SOFT MARKERS

During a routine anomaly scan, features may be identified within the fetus that are associated with but not diagnostic of other fetal problems, particularly karyotypic abnormalities. The first such finding reported was choroid plexus cysts, anechoic areas within the choroid plexus. Initially, these were thought to be completely benign (Chudleigh *et al.* 1984) but later accounts suggested an aneuploidy risk of up to 8%. With further

Table 3.3 Soft markers and associated fetal problems		
Soft marker	Incidence in obstetric population (%)	Quoted risk of potential fetal problems
Choroid plexus cyst	1	Trisomy 21: no increased risk if < 35 years Trisomy 18: > 40 years 1:200 Overall risk of aneuploidy if > 35 years 1:150
Echogenic bowel	1	Trisomy 21: 1.5% overall (less in younger women, higher with increased maternal age) Intrauterine growth restriction: 20% Cystic fibrosis: no increased risk in low-risk populations
Renal pelvis dilatation (5–8 mm)	3	Trisomy 21: 0–1%[a] Neonatal childhood nephropathy: 30%
Echogenic foci in heart	3–5	Trisomy 21: (0.002%); other markers almost always seen if trisomy 21 present
Isolated short femur length	~ 6	Trisomy 21: 2–0%

[a] 1% risk quoted from studies in selected populations

repeated studies in unselected or low risk populations, it was agreed that the risk of trisomy 18 or 21 in a fetus with isolated choroid plexus cyst was small, but more significant in women over 35 years of age. This huge swing in opinion over a relatively short period of time highlights the need for caution when interpreting new ultrasound features within the fetus. Other soft markers that have been identified include echogenic bowel, a short femur, strawberry-shaped skull, echogenic foci in the heart, renal pelvis dilatation and nuchal oedema. The potential fetal problems with which these soft markers have been linked are summarised in Table 3.3. It is important to remember that most pregnancies noted to have 'soft markers' have a completely normal outcome. Estimating the actual risk of these rare but associated problems in a fetus with soft markers remains an area of great debate. Table 3.3 also includes an estimate of these risks based on a range of reported reviews. In the absence of absolute risks, it is imperative that, within each department, standardised information is given to patients.

MISSED ANOMALIES: FALSE REASSURANCE

Some women who attend for ultrasound scan during pregnancy will give birth to a child with an abnormality. There are several reasons why this may occur. First, each department will have a set list of structures examined. Many units will not routinely look for a cleft lip and will not examine the outflow tracts of the heart. In this situation, the abnormality may be 'missed' because it does not fall into the list of structures to be evaluated. Second, abnormalities may not be diagnosed because they have not manifested themselves; for example, the diagnostic features of critical aortic stenosis and duodenal atresia may not be evident in the second trimester fetus. Likewise, the stomach may appear in an appropriate position at 18 weeks of gestation but be clearly seen within the chest cavity at 26 weeks due to a diaphragmatic hernia. Third, limitations in imaging, particularly in obese patients, may never be overcome, despite their having been scanned on several occasions, and abnormalities may be missed. Finally, as the RADIUS study demonstrated (Ewigman *et al*. 1993), abnormalities may not be recognised due to inadequately trained personnel and/or inappropriate machinery being used for the examination. For this reason the Royal College of Obstetricians and Gynaecologists introduced guidelines on training and equipment in early scans (RCOG 1997) and, more recently, specific recommendations for routine anomaly scanning in pregnancy (RCOG 2000).

Extract from the Recommendations of the RCOG (1997) Working Party on Ultrasound Screening for Fetal Abnormalities in Pregnancy

1. Women should positively opt in for a routine anomaly scan.

2. Written information should be available prior to the scan outlining the objectives and limitations of the scan. The detection rates for major abnormalities within the department concerned should be clearly defined.

3. Following diagnosis of an abnormality, staff should be available to discuss the implications of the findings and arrange any additional investigations or referrals required within 72 hours.

4. Detailed audit of the screening service should be ongoing and autopsies advised following termination of pregnancy to confirm antenatal findings.

5. Following termination of pregnancy, parents should be invited for a follow-up visit to discuss the results of any investigations, including post-mortem findings, and outline the risks for any future pregnancies.

6. Ultrasound examinations should only be conducted by appropriately trained personnel and should be conducted using an agreed protocol or checklist.

PARENTAL ANXIETY

There is little known about the psychological effects of routine anomaly scans on the prospective parents. Couples who have known other family members or friends to have had a child with an abnormality often describe a period of acute anxiety until the ultrasound examination is completed. For others, anxiety is generated during the examination when an abnormality, however minor, is identified. Anxiety is particularly intense when:

- the abnormality identified is not specific, e.g. mild renal pelvis dilatation, 'soft markers'
- the degree of handicap for the surviving child cannot be predicted, e.g. spina bifida
- decisions regarding termination of pregnancy require to be faced.

Support systems should be available within every department for such couples to help them work through and cope with the uncertainty of pregnancy or the issues involved with termination of pregnancy.

Conclusions

Routine anomaly scans in the second trimester are the most effective method to date for detecting structural fetal abnormalities. To ensure that the problems associated with a routine anomaly scan do not outweigh its benefits, patients and staff must be clear about the objectives and the limitations of such a scan. The RCOG recommendations outline how this may be achieved (see box on page 38). While improved imaging and first-trimester scans may well increase the detection rates of fetal anomalies, it should be stressed that fetal abnormality is but one cause of fetal morbidity and mortality and no pregnancy can be guaranteed a completely 'normal' outcome.

References

Boyd PA, Chamberlain P, Hicks NR. (1998) 6-year experience of prenatal diagnosis in an unselected population in Oxford, UK. *Lancet* **352**:577–81.

Braithwaite JM, Armstrong MA, Economides DL. (1996) The assessment of fetal anatomy at 12–13 weeks using transabdominal and transvaginal sonography. *Br J Obstet Gynaecol* **103**:82–5.

Chitty IS, Hunt GH, Moore J, Lobb MO. (1991) Effectiveness of routine ultrasonography in detecting fetal structural abnormalities in a low risk population. *BMJ*, **303**:1165–9.

Chudleigh P, Pearce M, Campbell S. (1984) The prenatal diagnosis of transient cysts of the fetal choroid plexus. *Prenat Diagn* **4**:135–7.

Ewigman BG, Crane JP, Frigoletto FD, LeFevre ML, Bain RP, McNellis D, RADIUS Study Group. (1993) Effect of prenatal ultrasound screening on perinatal outcome. *N Engl J Med*, **329**:821–7.

Luck CA. (1992) Value of routine ultrasound screening at 19 weeks: a four year study of 8849 deliveries. *BMJ* **304**:1474–8.

Royal College of Obstetricians and Gynaecologists. (1997) *Ultrasound Screening for Fetal Abnormalities: Report of the RCOG Working Party*. London: RCOG Press.

Royal College of Obstetricians and Gynaecologists. (2000) *Routine Ultrasound Screening in Pregnancy: Protocol, Standards and Training. Supplement to Ultrasound Screening for Fetal Abnormalities: Report of the RCOG Working Party*. London: RCOG Press.

Sharland G, Allan AD. (1992) Screening for congenital heart disease prenatally. Results of a 2-year study in the South East Thames Region. *Br J Obstet Gynaecol* **99**:220–5.

Shirley IM, Bottomley F, Robinson VP. (1992) Routine radiographerscreening for fetal abnormaliteis by ultrasound in an unselected low risk population. *Br J Radiol* **65**:564–9.

Whitlow BJ, Chatzipapas IK, Lazanakis ML, Kadir RA, Economides DL. (1999) The value of sonography in early pregnancy for the detection of fetal abnormalities in an unselected population. *Br J Obstet Gynaecol* **106**:929–36.

4 Fetal structural abnormalities

Introduction

Approximately 2% of births are affected by a single major structural abnormality (OPCS 1994). The frequency of structural anomaly is higher at conception but declines owing to the natural attrition rate associated with abnormal fetuses. The frequency with which the different body systems are affected is highlighted in Table 4.1. Congenital malformation has multiple aetiologies as illustrated in Table 4.2. As discussed in Chapter 3, antenatal diagnosis of fetal anomaly may have important implications for the subsequent management of the pregnancy. A comprehensive discussion of structural abnormalities is beyond the scope of this chapter, which should be viewed as an introduction to the subject.

Table 4.1 Frequency of structural malformations

Body system	Cases per 1000 births (n)
Central nervous	10
Cardiovascular	8
Renal	4
Limbs	2
Other	6
Total	30

Table 4.2 Aetiology of congenital malformation

Aetiology	Type (%)
Idiopathic	60.0
Multifactorial	20.0
Single gene disorder	7.5
Chromosomal	6.0
Maternal illness	3.0
Congenital infection	2.0
Drugs, X-ray, alcohol	1.5

Table 4.3	Risk factors for neural tube defects
Factor	Example
Elevated maternal serum α-fetoprotein	
Family history	Risk 1:25 if one affected parent or sibling Risk 1:10 if two affected siblings
Maternal disorder	Diabetes mellitus, epilepsy
Drugs	Sodium valproate, phenytoin, carbamazepine
Chromosomal abnormalities	Trisomy 18, trisomy 13
Single gene mutations	Meckel–Gruber syndrome (autosomal recessive)

Central nervous system

Neural tube defects comprise anencephaly (40%), spina bifida (55%) and encephalocele (5%). Risk factors for these conditions are shown in Table 4.3. There is geographical variation in the frequency of neural tube defects, the west of Scotland and Ireland having the highest incidence in Great Britain. The birth incidence of these conditions has fallen, with an estimated two cases per 1000 in the west of Scotland. The reason for this decline in birth frequency is unknown and is not simply due to the option of termination of an affected pregnancy.

Screening programmes for neural tube defects were introduced in the 1970s. They rely on estimation of maternal serum α-FP concentrations and results are expressed as multiples of the median. Individual screening programmes employ a cut-off point that maximises detection of affected pregnancies while maintaining an acceptable false positive rate. Screening is performed between 15 and 21 weeks of gestation, the optimum time being 16–18 weeks, and in the west of Scotland an α-FP level of ≥ 2 MOM will detect 100% of cases of anencephaly and 80% of cases of open spina bifida. The diagnostic test following a positive screening test result for neural tube defects is ultrasound, which will detect 100% of cases of anencephaly and 98% of cases of open spina bifida.

ANENCEPHALY

Anencephaly is a lethal condition in which there is absence of the cerebral hemispheres and most of the cranial vault. This results in prominent orbits and the typical 'frog-like' appearance on transabdominal ultrasound (Figure 4.1).

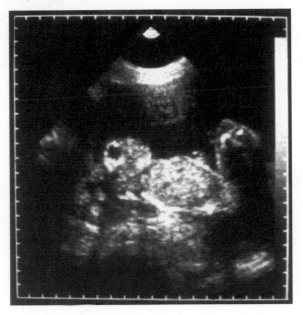

Figure 4.1 Anencephaly: the cranial vault is absent and the orbits are prominent producing the characteristic 'frog-like' appearance

SPINA BIFIDA

Spina bifida results from failure of closure of the neural groove, a process that is normally complete by 28 days post-conception. The lesion may be open (Figure 4.2: Plate 1) or closed, the latter having a skin covering. Closed lesions are usually small, α-FP levels are not increased and antenatal detection by ultrasound is frequently not possible. In open lesions, the bony spine and overlying skin are disrupted and a bulging meningeal membrane is apparent. If neural tissue is present within the sac it is termed a myelomeningocele. The lumbosacral area is most commonly affected. There may be associated cranial features including the Arnold–Chiari malformation, which generally results in obstructive hydrocephalus. The 'lemon' and 'banana' signs describe the ultrasound features of the Arnold–Chiari malformation; the former refers to scalloping of the frontal bones resulting in a lemon-shaped head (Figure 4.3) and the latter describes the shape of the cerebellum owing to caudal displacement. The degree of handicap can be difficult to predict in the antenatal period. The extent of physical handicap depends in part on the site and size of the lesion, and there may be gross paralysis of the lower limbs with bladder and bowel dysfunction. Intelligence can be normal but it is impossible to predict this *in utero*. Termination is one of the options

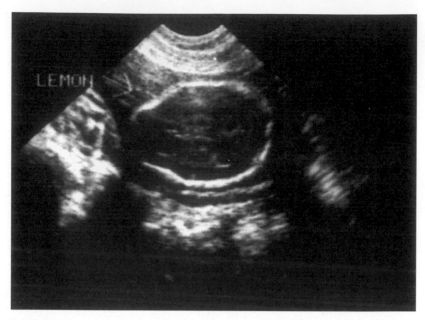

Figure 4.3 'Lemon' sign; scalloping of the frontal bones gives the skull a lemon shape

available. Those couples choosing to continue with the pregnancy should have access to multidisciplinary counselling and delivery should take place in a unit with a neonatal surgical department.

ENCEPHALOCELE

Encephalocele accounts for approximately 5% of neural tube defects. The lesion is most commonly occipital (75%) and intracranial contents protrude through a bony defect in the skull (Figure 4.4: Plate 1). It is important to demonstrate a bony defect in order to differentiate encephalocele from other causes of soft tissue swelling, e.g. cystic hygroma or hydrops. Up to 15% of encephaloceles have a coexistent spina bifida lesion.

ADDITIONAL ANOMALIES

Detection of a structural abnormality on ultrasound should always lead to a thorough search for additional anomalies, since their presence can alter the diagnosis, management and implications for a future pregnancy. For example, a fetus with an isolated neural tube defect may be managed entirely differently from a fetus with a neural tube defect and an exomphalos, which could indicate trisomy 18, a lethal condition.

Table 4.4 Mechanisms resulting in hydrocephalus	
Mechanism	*Aetiology*
Obstruction to outflow, e.g. aquaductal stenosis	Genetic, e.g. X-linked recessive, infection, e.g. cytomegalovirus, toxoplasmosis, syphilis, teratogenic, haemorrhage, tumours/mass lesions
Impaired cerebrospinal fluid resorption	
Overproduction of cerebrospinal fluid	
Underdevelopment/destruction of cortical tissue	

Alternatively a neural tube defect and polycystic kidneys suggest a diagnosis of Meckel–Gruber syndrome, which has a recurrence risk of 1:4, in contrast to a recurrence risk of 1:25 for an isolated lesion. Karyotyping may therefore be appropriate in the presence of multiple defects.

Preconceptional folic acid supplementation, 0.4 mg daily, reduces the incidence of neural tube defects. Women who have had a previously affected pregnancy or who are taking anticonvulsants should take a higher daily dose (4 mg).

HYDROCEPHALUS

Hydrocephalus is an increase in the intracranial content of cerebrospinous fluid, which results in ventriculomegaly. The mechanisms leading to hydrocephalus are detailed in Table 4.4, obstruction being the most common aetiology. Ultrasound diagnosis relies on demonstrating an increase in the size of some or all of the ventricles. The condition is referred to as isolated hydrocephalus provided that there are no other structural abnormalities. However, approximately one-third of cases have additional anomalies, the most common being spina bifida, and about 10% of fetuses with hydrocephalus will have a karyotypic abnormality.

Cardiovascular system

Congenital heart disease (CHD) accounts for 20% of neonatal deaths and 50% of deaths arising from congenital abnormality (Hoffman and Christianson 1978). The livebirth frequency of different types of CHD is given in Table 4.5. Risk factors for CHD are illustrated in Table 4.6. However, the majority of babies with CHD will be delivered to women with no identifiable risk factors, which highlights the limitations of 'high-risk' population screening in the antenatal detection of CHD. Incorporating

Table 4.5 Distribution of congenital heart disease in liveborn affected infants (adapted with permission from Hoffman and Christianson 1978)

Lesion	Frequency (%)
Ventricular septal defect	30.3
Pulmonary stenosis	7.4
Atrial septal defect (secundum)	6.7
Aortic stenosis	5.2
Tetralogy of Fallot	5.1
Transposition of great vessels	4.7
Atrioventricular septal defect	3.2
Hypoplastic left-heart syndrome	1.3
Truncus arteriosus	1.0

Table 4.6 Risk factors for congenital heart disease

Type of risk	Factor
Familial	One affected sibling recurrence risk 2–5% Two affected siblings 10–15%
Maternal:	
Medical conditions	Diabetes, systemic lupus erythematosus, phenylketonuria
Drugs	Anticonvulsants, lithium, alcohol, amphetamines, heroin, cocaine, thalidomide
Infections	Rubella, toxoplasmosis, cytomegalovirus
Fetal:	
Extracardiac anomalies	Hydrocephalus, Dandy–Walker malformation, oesophageal atresia, exomphalos, diaphragmatic hernia, renal agenesis, single umbilical artery
Non-immune hydrops	
Fetal arrhythmias	
Symmetrical IUGR	
Polyhydramnios	
Chromosomal abnormalities	Trisomy 21, trisomy 18, trisomy 13, 45X

Table 4.7 Cardiac anomalies detected according to type of ultrasound examination

Four-chamber view	Echocardiography
Hypoplastic left-heart syndrome	Tetralogy of Fallot
Ebstein's anomaly	Transposition of great vessels
Atrioventricular canal malformation	Common truncus arteriosus
	Atrial or ventricular septal defects
	Pulmonary and aortic stenosis

the four-chamber view is the proposed method to improve the sensitivity of level I scans in screening for CHD. In the most experienced hands only 40–50% of cardiac anomalies are amenable to detection employing this view alone, and therefore this level of screening reduces the risk of CHD by at most 50%, a fact of which women should be aware. Anomalies that can be detected from the four-chamber view alone are detailed in Table 4.7. Detection of other cardiac anomalies requires the more extended examination of fetal echocardiography, for which sensitivities of 88.5% have been reported (Stumpflen *et al.* 1996). It is important to recognise that not all cardiac abnormalities can be detected antenatally.

EXTRACARDIAC ANOMALIES

Up to 44% of congenital heart lesions are associated with anomalies in one or more body systems (Wallgren *et al.* 1978). Examples are given in Table 4.6. Extracardiac anomalies are more frequent with certain cardiac lesions, e.g. ventricular septal defect, tetralogy of Fallot and coarctation of the aorta. There is a strong association between CHD and aneuploidy. Chromosomal abnormalities that are commonly reported include trisomies 21, 18 and 13 and Turner syndrome. Certain combinations of anomalies should increase suspicion regarding a specific syndrome or chromosomal abnormality (Table 4.8). Certain cardiac anomalies are more frequently associated with aneuploidy, such as atrioventricular septal defect and double outlet right ventricle, and the presence of additional extracardiac anomalies further increases the risk. Karyotyping, after appropriate counselling, should be considered when a cardiac defect is detected antenatally by ultrasound.

A detailed discussion of individual cardiac defects is beyond the scope of this chapter. However, a few specific features are worth consideration. Hypoplastic left-heart syndrome (HLHS) was once viewed as a universally fatal condition. Advances in surgical expertise have resulted in five-year survival figures for surgically corrected HLHS in the region of 70%

Table 4.8 Examples of structure defects associated with chromosomal abnormalities

Chromosomal defects	Associated malformations
Trisomy 21	Atrioventricular canal defect Duodenal atresia
Trisomy 18	Ventricular septal defect Exomphalos Micrognathia
Trisomy 13	Ventricular septal defect Holoprosencephaly Facial cleft
Turner syndrome	Coarctation of the aorta

provided that there are no complicating factors or extracardiac anomalies (O'Kelly and Bove 1997). Ebstein's anomaly, in which the primary defect is displacement of the tricuspid valve, is associated with cardiac failure *in utero* in approximately 50% of cases. Atrioventricular septal defects are associated with trisomy 21 in 50% of cases and karyotyping should therefore be offered. Ventricular septal defects are frequently part of more complex congenital heart disease and, if extracardiac anomalies are present, a chromosomal abnormality should be suspected. Cardiac defects *per se* are not associated with intrauterine growth restriction (IUGR). However, if there is haemodynamic compromise during fetal life, IUGR may occur. Aortic stenosis is the lesion most commonly associated with IUGR.

Table 4.9 Features of gastroschisis and exomphalos

Factor	Gastroschisis	Exomphalos
Site of defect	Paraumbilical (right)	Umbilical
Cord insertion	Left of defect	Apex of sac
Covering membrane	No	Yes
Maternal serum α-fetoprotein	Raised	May be normal
Additional anomalies	Rare (< 10%)	30–70% (central nervous system, cardiac, renal)
Chromosomal abnormalities	Rare (< 1%)	Up to 60%
Karyotyping	Rarely indicated	Should be offered

Gastrointestinal system

The common anterior abdominal wall defects comprise gastroschisis and exomphalos. They are both amenable to antenatal diagnosis and, provided that they are isolated defects, the prognosis following early neonatal surgery is excellent for each condition (at least 80% survival). Table 4.9 illustrates the differing features of the two conditions. The incidence of gastroschisis is approximately one in 2500–3000 live births. There is a defect in the abdominal wall to the right side of the umbilicus through which gastrointestinal contents, usually bowel, herniate (Figure 4.5: Plate 2). Free loops of bowel are seen floating in the amniotic cavity on ultrasound examination. In contrast, exomphalos (Figure 4.6) is a

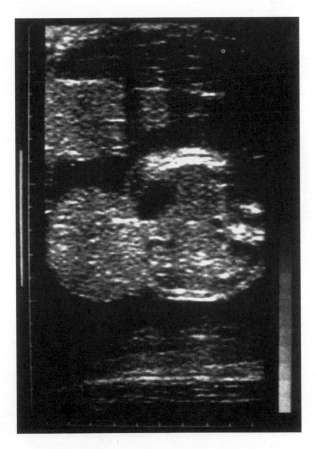

Figure 4.6 Exomphalos: ultrasound cross-section of the fetal abdomen with sac of herniated contents on the left

midline defect in which the herniated contents are covered by a membrane and the umbilical cord inserts into the apex of the lesion. The incidence is approximately one in 5000 live births. As indicated in Table 4.9, exomphalos is associated with chromosomal and additional structural abnormalities, whereas these are rare in gastroschisis. Management involves excluding additional anomalies and offering karyotyping in cases of exomphalos. Serial estimation of fetal growth should be performed, accepting the limitations of abdominal circumference measurements in these conditions. Close fetal surveillance is required towards term and delivery should be at term unless indicated earlier by other features. There is no evidence to support routine caesarean section for these conditions and, provided that the presentation is cephalic, vaginal delivery should be aimed for. Delivery should take place in a centre with access to a neonatal surgical unit.

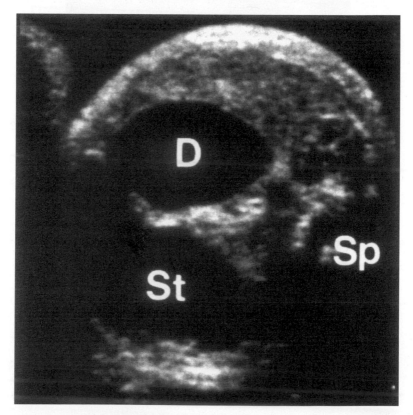

Figure 4.7 Duodenal atresia: cross-section through the fetal abdomen demonstrating 'double bubble'; D = duodenum; St = stomach; Sp = spine

Body stalk anomaly is a rare abdominal wall defect (one in 14000 births) in which there is no umbilical cord and the herniated abdominal contents are attached directly to the placenta. Other anomalies are frequently present, including neural tube defects and lower limb abnormalities. It is a lethal condition and termination of pregnancy should be offered.

Congenital diaphragmatic hernia has an incidence of 0.35 per 1000 births in the UK. It is most commonly a posterolateral lesion located on the left side (80%). It is associated with additional structural anomalies (CVS, neural tube defects and exomphalos) and the risk of aneuploidy is 10–20%. Karyotyping should therefore be offered. Demonstration of fluid-filled bowel at the level of the four-chamber view of the heart on ultrasound is diagnostic, although it is a diagnosis that can easily be missed, since there can be free movement of bowel through the defect. Favourable prognostic features are a left-sided hernia and diagnosis after 24 weeks of gestation. Prognosis can, however, be difficult to predict in the antenatal period.

Duodenal atresia occurs in one in 10000 live births. It is an isolated defect in only 50% of cases and, since up to 30% are associated with trisomy 21, karyotyping should be offered. The ultrasound appearance is of a 'double bubble' due to the stomach and dilated duodenum proximal to the atresia (Figure 4.7). Polyhydramnios is often present.

Renal tract abnormalities

In the context of renal tract abnormalities oligohydramnios indicates one of the following:

- absent kidneys
- outflow tract obstruction
- deteriorating renal function secondary to an intrinsic renal problem.

Table 4.10 Classification of cystic renal disease

Type	Potter classification	Inheritance
Infantile polycystic kidneys	Type 1	Autosomal recessive
Multicystic kidney disease	Type 2	Usually sporadic; if component of Meckel–Gruber syndrome, autosomal recessive
Adult polycystic kidney disease	Type 3	Autosomal dominant
Cystic renal dysplasia	Type 4	Sporadic

Bilateral renal agenesis is a uniformly fatal condition with an incidence of approximately one in 3000 births. It is one of the differential diagnoses of oligohydramnios detected at a second-trimester scan. It is a diagnosis that is difficult to make because visualisation of the anatomy is restricted owing to oligo/anhydramnios. Amnioinfusion can be helpful to confirm the absence of kidneys and bladder filling. It is generally a sporadic condition but can be associated with other malformations. Termination of pregnancy is one of the management options.

Cystic disease of the kidneys is classified into four types (Table 4.10). Infantile polycystic kidneys are bilaterally enlarged with a bright echogenic appearance on ultrasound. There is a spectrum of severity but, when the diagnosis is made antenatally, the prognosis is generally guarded. Adult polycystic kidney disease is by definition rarely diagnosed *in utero*. Multicystic kidney disease may be bilateral, unilateral or involve only a segment of the kidney. The cysts are peripheral and may be multiple, varying in size. If unilateral, abnormalities of the contralateral kidney are present in up to 50% of cases. Finally, renal dysplasia secondary to obstruction will lead to hyperechogenic kidneys on ultrasound. In this situation the kidneys may be small or enlarged.

Renal tract obstruction can occur at any level from the renal pelvis to the urethra and may be unilateral or bilateral. Pelviureteric obstruction is the most common cause of hydronephrosis. It is more common in males and is unilateral in 70% of cases. A measurement of the renal pelvis in the transverse plane of greater than 5 mm before 28 weeks of gestation and greater than 10 mm beyond 28 weeks of gestation requires surveillance. Additional structural abnormalities may be present and the condition is also associated with trisomy 21, particularly if bilateral. Obstruction at the level of the urethra, secondary to posterior urethral valves, is the most common cause of bladder dilatation. It occurs almost exclusively in males. Back pressure leads to bilateral hydroureters and hydronephrosis. Not only do the kidneys become dysplastic as a result, but growth and development of the lungs may also be compromised owing to oligohydramnios. The condition is amenable to *in utero* therapy (vesico-amniotic shunt), but adequate renal function must be demonstrated first by serial urinary electrolyte analysis, and the outlook with a functioning shunt is difficult to predict.

Antenatal ultrasound is an indirect method of assessing renal function and relies on measurement of amniotic fluid volume. When a fetus is identified with a renal problem additional abnormalities should be sought. If an isolated problem exists, serial scans are required to monitor renal tract architecture and liquor volume. The timing of delivery will be indicated by these parameters.

Table 4.11 Features of common skeletal dysplasias

Type	Mode of inheritance	Severity
Thanatophoric dysplasia	Sporadic	Lethal
Osteogenesis imperfecta type II	Heterogeneous	Lethal
Achondrogenesis	Autosomal recessive	Lethal
Achondroplasia	Autosomal dominant, mainly new mutations	Normal lifespan

Skeletal system

Skeletal dysplasias are a heterogeneous group of disorders that account for approximately 1% of perinatal deaths. Only the four most common dysplasias will be mentioned. Table 4.11 summarises some of the features of these conditions. Thanatophoric dysplasia is the most common. It is characterised by short proximal bones and a hypoplastic 'bell-shaped' chest on ultrasound. Osteogenesis imperfecta is a collagen disorder that results in increased bone fragility. Type II is the most frequently encountered form and it is amenable to antenatal diagnosis. Fractures may occur *in utero*, leading to a bowed or angulated appearance of the long bones. One characteristic ultrasound feature is indentation of the fetal skull secondary to pressure from the ultrasound transducer.

In achondrogenesis, there is severe limb shortening and hypomineralisation. Two types are described, according to the degree of abnormal ossification of the spine. Achondroplasia is characterised by short proximal limb bones (rhizomelia), a large head and a depressed nasal bridge. While inheritance is autosomal dominant most cases are the result of a new mutation. Skeletal dysplasias are associated with hydramnios and, although amenable to antenatal diagnosis, detection of long-bone growth abnormalities may not be possible until the third trimester.

Conclusions

Detection of a fetal structural anomaly should prompt a number of responses. First, a thorough structural survey must be performed to identify the presence of additional anomalies that can affect diagnosis and management and have implications for future pregnancies. Karyotyping may be indicated and appropriate counselling is essential. Discussion with a multidisciplinary team is often required to help couples make an informed decision about the subsequent management of the pregnancy. Not only is this important to help them understand the nature of the condition, it also prepares them for events that will take place in the immediate neonatal period and indeed in the long term. In certain circumstances it will be appropriate to transfer care to a tertiary referral centre where there is access to neonatal surgeons. When the outlook for the pregnancy is poor and termination is the chosen option, the importance of postmortem examination should be discussed, to ensure that as much information as possible is available for counselling regarding future pregnancies.

References

Hoffman JI, Christianson R. (1978) Congenital heart disease in a cohort of 19,502 births with long-term follow-up. *Am J Cardiol* **42**:641–7.

O'Kelly SW, Bove EL. (1997) Hypoplastic left heart syndrome. Terminal care is not the only option. *BMJ* **314**:87–8.

Office of Population Censuses and Surveys. (1994) London: HMSO.

Stumpflen I, Stumpflen A, Wimmer M, Bernaschek G. (1996) Effect of detailed fetal echocardiography as part of routine prenatal ultrasonographic screening on detection of congenital heart disease. *Lancet* **348**:854–7.

Wallgren EI, Landtman B, Rapola J. (1978) Extracardiac malformations associated with congenital heart disease. *Eur J Cardiol* **7**: 15–24.

5 Fetal therapy

Historical aspects

Treatment of the fetus *in utero* has been a possibility for obstetricians since the 1960s. This was a time when the dawn of a new branch of medicine, perinatal medicine, became a reality through the contributions of obstetricians such as Professor Ian Donald in Glasgow and Dr AW Liley in New Zealand. Their research on the development of ultrasound and amniocentesis in rhesus sensitisation enabled doctors to treat the fetus as a patient. Since then, other milestones in the creation of this branch of medicine have been Professor GC Liggins' work in the 1970s on the maternal administration of corticosteroids to prevent respiratory distress syndrome and the practical and laboratory genetic techniques for prenatal diagnosis in the first trimester of pregnancy throughout the 1980s. The key to the success of attempts at fetal diagnosis and therapy has been the continued improvement in fetal imaging techniques, mainly with high-resolution ultrasound techniques and the use of ultra-fast magnetic resonance imaging (MRI). In the future, rapid progress is likely to be made in real time three-dimensional ultrasound procedures and, together with advances in minimal-access surgical techniques, the concept of providing true fetal treatment is a real possibility in the years ahead.

The main clinical areas of focus as regards potential fetal therapy have been prematurity, IUGR, fetal malformations and specific genetic conditions. The main types of fetal therapy that were introduced include preventive therapy, transplacental treatment, perinatal management of the fetus with a malformation and invasive fetal procedures.

PREVENTIVE THERAPY

This involves public health education giving general advice on maternal health and diet with a specific focus on smoking cessation and limitation of alcohol intake during pregnancy (RCOG 1999).

Certain fetal malformations, such as neural tube defects, warrant specific consideration. The birth prevalence of neural tube defects varies geographically, from less than one per 1000 to over four per 1000 (Little and Elwood 1992). Women who have had one infant with a neural tube defect have a risk of recurrence some ten-fold greater than women in general, about 3–4%. It has been clearly shown that the majority of defects can be prevented by increasing maternal folic acid intake over the time of conception and through the first 12 weeks of pregnancy (MRC Vitamin Research Group 1991). The recommended supplementary dose of folic acid is 400 µg in addition to the average dietary intake of 0.2 mg daily. Health authorities, hospital and primary care trusts are trying to increase public awareness of this important preventive strategy through promotional materials in GP surgeries, hospital clinics and in pharmacists' shops.

A higher dose of 5 mg daily is recommended for women with insulin-dependent diabetes, epilepsy and women who have had a previous pregnancy affected with a neural tube defect.

Other prepregnancy advice, such as avoidance of drugs and potential teratogens, should be widely given, as should specific measures such as rubella vaccination to those at risk and strict control of the blood sugar in women with insulin-dependent diabetes.

Fetal therapy in women who have inborn errors of metabolism can be considered in a number of ways. The maternal metabolic disorder may be the primary disease and an adverse fetal effect secondary. Optimal maternal care is then required for the wellbeing of both the mother and her fetus. This is the case in maternal phenylketonuria (PKU) and Wilson's disease, where the fetus is the passive victim of the maternal metabolic derangement. In these conditions, the primary goal of maternal therapy is to optimise the fetal environment to minimise the risk of fetal damage in an otherwise unaffected fetus.

Indirect (transplacental) fetal therapy

MEDICAL TREATMENT AND FETAL PHARMOKINETICS

The mechanism for medical fetal therapy involves the transplacental passage of substances via the maternal circulation. This chiefly involves administration of a drug, hormone or vitamin to the mother. Drugs mainly move across the placenta by simple diffusion but the process is dependent on the chemical properties and concentration gradients of the free drug. Drug transfer is greater in late gestation, but pathological conditions causing inflammation, hypoxia vascular degeneration or separation of the placenta can affect uteroplacental blood flow and thus transfer of the drug. Like the liver, the placenta is capable of drug biotransformation and some drugs may only cross the placenta after this has occurred. For most drugs that cross the placenta, fetal levels reach 50–100% of maternal serum concentrations. However, once the levels reach steady state, fetal serum levels can be higher than maternal levels. It is the total time exposed to a

PLATE 1

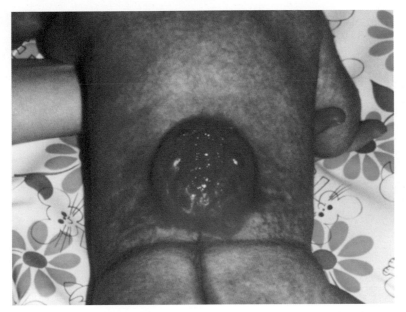

Figure 4.2 Open spina bifida

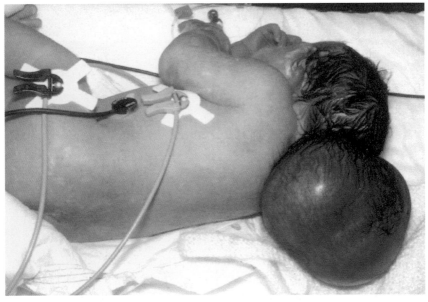

Figure 4.4 Occipital encephalocele

PLATE 2

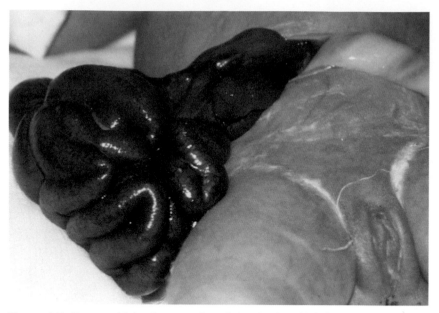

Figure 4.5 Gastroschisis: the anterior abdominal wall defect is to the right of the umbilical cord

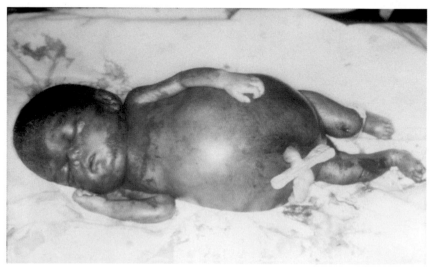

Figure 5.4b Hydrops fetalis

PLATE 3

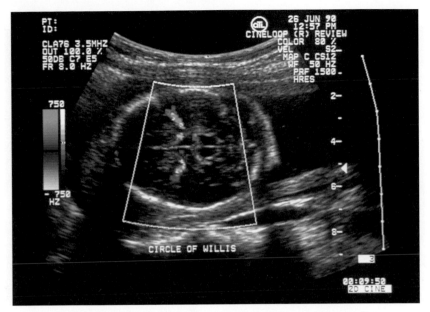

Figure 5.6a Measurement of cerebral artery peak systolic velocity: Doppler ultrasound

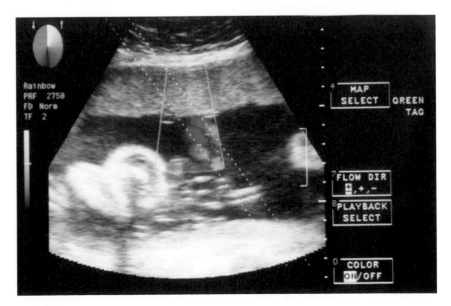

Figure 5.7a Intravascular transfusion

PLATE 4

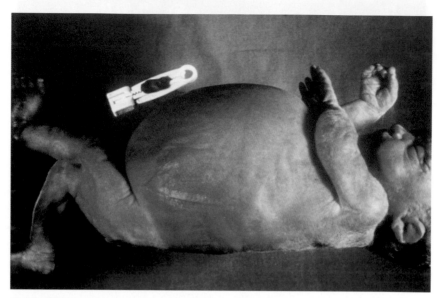

Figure 5.12 A fetus with 'prune belly' syndrome

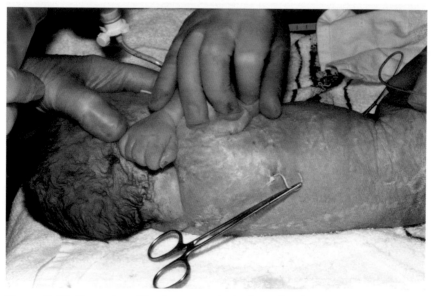

Figure 5.15 Neonate with pleuroamniotic shunt in place

PLATE 5

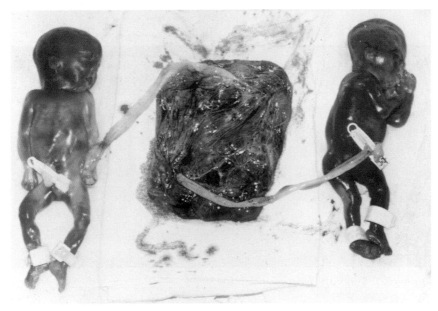

Figure 5.16 Twin-to-twin transfusion syndrome; donor left, recipient right

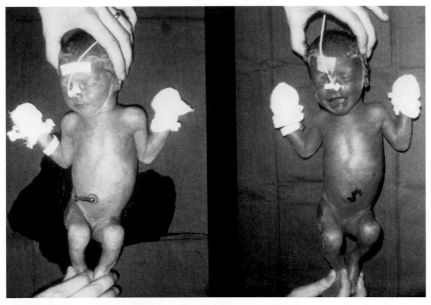

Figure 5.17 Surviving fetuses of twin-to-twin transfusion syndrome; donor left, recipient right

PLATE 6

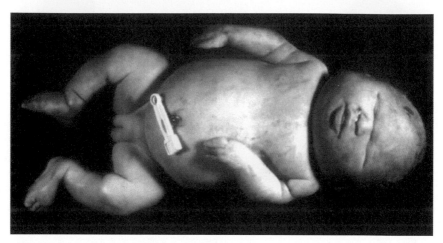

Figure 6.1 Stillborn hydropic neonate

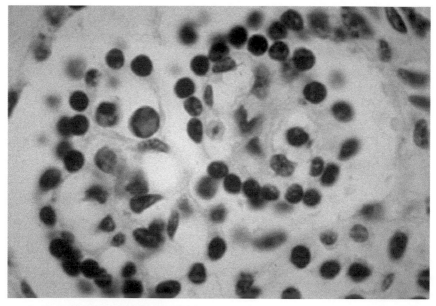

Figure 6.6 Human parvovirus B19

PLATE 7

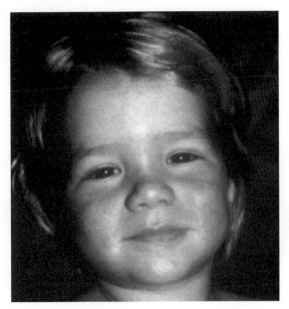

Figure 6.7 Slapped cheek syndrome

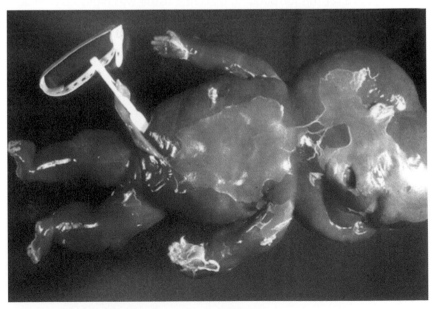

Figure 6.8 Hydropic intrauterine death due to parvovirus B19

PLATE 8

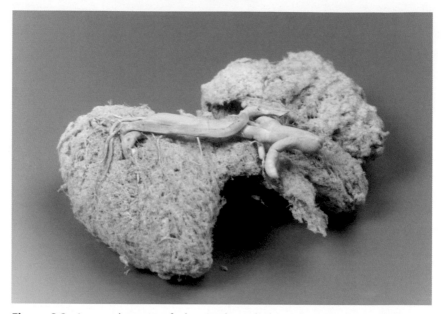

Figure 8.2 A vascular cast of placental cotyledon: the vessels supplying a cotyledon were injected with plastic to form a mould of the vessel network; once set the surrounding placental tissue was digested with acid solution, leaving the plastic mould of the vessels within the villi; the extensive network of vessels can be clearly seen and can then be examined by scanning microscopy

drug and its metabolites that is more important than the rate of transplacental transport. In view of the fact that fetal systems are not fully developed, the excretion of drugs is much slower than in the adult. The main routes of elimination involve the placenta and fetal urine. In early pregnancy, the primary route of elimination is by placental transfer to the maternal circulation, whereas in later gestation drugs are eliminated into the amniotic fluid via the fetal kidneys.

CONGENITAL ADRENAL HYPERPLASIA

Congenital adrenal hyperplasia (CAH) was the first example of an inborn error of metabolism inherited by the fetus that can be treated *in utero* with prevention of the malformation as the primary goal. This disorder has been linked to chromosome 6. The clinical spectrum of disease associated with CAH ranges from the life-threatening wasting variety to mild virilisation in males or ambiguous genitalia in females. Prominent clitoromegaly with labial fusion can lead to incorrect gender assignment at birth.

Since CAH is an autosomal recessive condition, and only the females will be affected by the anomaly, the birth defect risk is one in eight. Virilisation of the female fetus may occur during weeks 10–16 of gestation, and therefore preventive *in utero* therapy needs to be started prior to the determination of gender or disease status. This can be achieved by suppressing the fetal adrenal gland by maternal administration of dexamethasone. It has been recommended that maternal dexamethasone therapy be initiated as early as five weeks of gestation using a dose of 20 µg/kg per day (Forest and David 1992). At ten weeks of gestation, CVS should be undertaken to determine the fetal sex and whether the fetus is affected using DNA analysis. If the fetus is unaffected or if an affected male fetus is discovered, maternal dexamethasone therapy can be stopped. If the fetus is an affected female, maternal therapy should be continued until delivery. Despite these measures, one-third of these neonates still exhibit some degree of virilisation.

FETAL DYSRHYTHMIAS

The majority of disturbances of fetal cardiac rhythm are noted either incidentally during auscultation of the fetal heart or during an ultrasound examination. The type of arrhythmia can be established using fetal M-mode echocardiography, and duplex-pulsed and colour Doppler (Figures 5.1 and 6.4).

The most common fetal dysrhythmia is supraventricular tachycardia (SVT) followed by atrial flutter. SVT is most often caused by reciprocating or atrioventricular re-entrant tachycardia. The ventricular rate is always

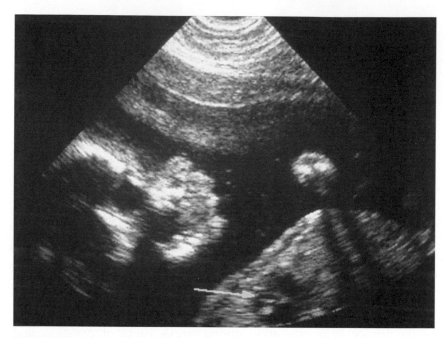

Figure 5.1 Fetal arrhythmia

rapid (240–260 bpm) and can lead to fetal hydrops. The need for fetal therapy is based upon a number of factors including gestational age, presence or absence of hydrops and the estimated duration of the tachycardia. Immature fetuses with hydrops are thus the most obvious candidates for anti-arrythmic treatment. The primary aim is to convert the rhythm back to normal *in utero* and to deliver the fetus in normal sinus rhythm at or near term (Simpson and Sharland 1998).

In SVT, digoxin is usually favoured for the non-hydropic fetus and flecainide for the hydropic fetus because of its better passage across the placenta. Maternal oral digoxin therapy is successful in approximately 60% of cases. The dose required is 0.5–1.0 mg daily. Flecainide is given at a dose of 100 mg twice daily. Fetuses that do not respond to either of these drugs may be candidates for direct fetal therapy in an attempt to achieve medical cardioversion of SVT using adenosine directly injected into the fetal umbilical or hepatic vein (Blanch *et al.* 1994).

Non-hydropic cases can be treated as outpatients, whereas hydropic cases require inpatient treatment. Evaluation and treatment should be performed in a tertiary fetal medicine centre. However, unless obstetric complications occur and the rhythm disturbance fails to respond to treatment, local delivery can be considered (Simpson 2000).

The types of rhythm disturbance causing fetal bradycardia include sinus bradycardia, blocked atrial ectopic beats and complete heart block. Examination using M-mode and Doppler echocardiography aids the differentiation. Atrial ectopic beats usually resolve spontaneously and therefore reassuring counselling is recommended. Fetuses with complete heart block should have a detailed cardiac ultrasound examination to look for evidence of associated CHD, and the mother should be checked for the presence of maternal autoantibodies, namely anti-SSA/Ro and anti-SSB/La. The detection of such antibodies is important, since there is potential fetal therapy in the form of maternal dexamethasone 4 mg daily. This has had limited success in a small number of cases (Copel *et al.* 1994). When fetal hydrops is present, the prognosis is poor and has not been improved by fetal therapy with agents such as salbutamol and direct fetal pacing. Fetuses with complete heart block should be delivered in a tertiary fetal medicine centre with easy access to a paediatric cardiology service.

Invasive fetal therapy

ULTRASOUND-GUIDED

The continuing improvements in ultrasound technology have permitted the fetal medicine specialist to examine the fetus in a similar way to other medical practitioners examining extrauterine patients. A variety of investigations can be undertaken and, in certain conditions, direct fetal treatment can be instigated in an attempt to improve the neonatal prognosis. All these developments involve multidisciplinary teamwork, which begins with detailed counselling prior to any planned intervention. In view of the complexities of such cases, invasive fetal therapy is usually performed in specialised tertiary referral centres where couples can be counselled and receive treatment from the members of the multidisciplinary perinatal team.

Prior to embarking on fetal therapy, a detailed assessment of both the maternal and fetal condition is required. The views and wishes of the prospective parents are entirely respected. Factors such as the need to exclude chromosomal abnormalities will be discussed prior to embarking on fetal therapy. The advantages and disadvantages of proposed therapies need to be discussed in great detail and in certain circumstances other members of the perinatal team will be involved. This will permit the parents to be fully aware of the potential neonatal prognosis and whether alternative strategies may offer other management options. It is crucial that such discussions take place in an unhurried, calm environment and that the parents are given ample time to ask questions and meet with other members of the perinatal group.

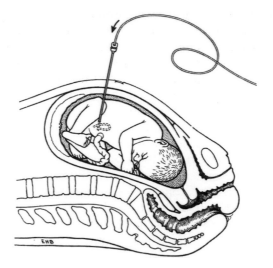

Figure 5.2 Intraperitoneal transfusion

INTRAVASCULAR TRANSFUSION FOR RHESUS DISEASE

Intrauterine transfusion was the original fetal therapy described by Liley in the 1960s. He described intraperitoneal transfusion via a catheter placed under fluoroscopic control into the fetal peritoneal cavity (Figure 5.2). Since then, there have been continued advances in this area of fetal therapy and the contribution of these procedures to the reduction of perinatal mortality due to Rh disease is illustrated in Figure 5.3.

A number of factors are taken into consideration when deciding upon the likely need of, and timing of, fetal blood transfusion. Maternal past obstetric history and neonatal history of top-up or exchange transfusion are both important since, if a subsequent pregnancy is affected, this is likely to occur at an earlier gestation. Maternal antibody quantification gives an indication of the progression of disease with the trend in rise of antibody levels being as important as a fixed cut-off level. Ultrasound surveillance to detect early signs of fetal hydrops (Figure 5.4a and Figure 5.4b: Plate 2) is important. Amniocentesis has traditionally been the next line of investigation following a rise in maternal antibodies. This technique allows measurement of the bilirubin concentration (Delta OD450) in amniotic fluid and gives an indirect estimate of fetal haemolysis. The level is plotted on the Liley curve (Figure 5.5) and this gives an estimation of risk depending upon which Liley zone the level corresponds to. Values for OD450 in the lower zone indicated a fetus with mild or no haemolytic disease while those in the upper zone indicated severe haemolytic disease with fetal death probable in 7–10 days. The Liley curve became the cornerstone of management for the pregnant patient with red cell alloimmunisation. However, in recent years there has been a loss of faith in amniocentesis as a useful tool for predicting fetal disease, especially at early gestations. Amniocentesis also carries the risk of aggravating maternal sensitisation and therefore the role of non-invasive tests has been explored.

Middle cerebral artery peak systolic velocity measurement is one such technique. The underlying theory is that the anaemic fetus has a reduced blood viscosity and increased cardiac output, both of which lead to a

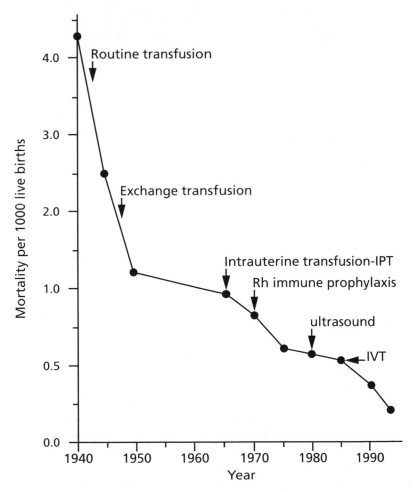

Figure 5.3 Developments in the management of rhesus disease; IPT = intraperitoneal transfusion; IVT = intravascular transfusion; Rh = rhesus

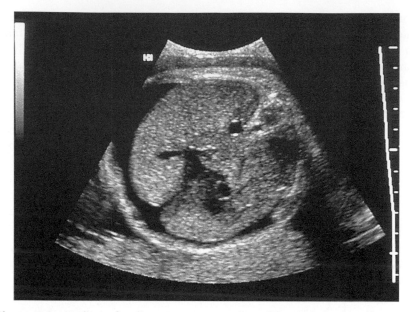

Figure 5.4a Hydrops fetalis: transverse section of fetal abdomen showing fetal ascites

measurable increase in peak systolic velocity (PSV) assessed by Doppler ultrasound (Figure 5.6a: Plate 3 and Figure 5.6b). Current evidence indicates that a PSV of greater than 1.5 MOM has 100% sensitivity in the prediction of moderate to severe anaemia (Mari *et al.* 2000), and it is starting to gain acceptance in clinical practice.

If intrauterine transfusion is deemed necessary, this should be performed in a tertiary referral centre experienced in the technique. The patient must be counselled regarding the nature of the procedure, the requirement for repeated transfusions and the potential complications.

Intrauterine transfusion is an aseptic technique carried out under ultrasound guidance. The patient is fasted, sedated and given antibiotics to cover the procedure. Steroids are given to promote pulmonary maturity once fetal viability is reached. The intravascular route has superseded the intraperitoneal route, which was the technique used for the first intrauterine transfusions. While the technique is simpler than an intravascular transfusion, the red cells have to be absorbed from the peritoneal cavity into the fetal circulation and hence the response to treatment is delayed. In current clinical practice intraperitoneal transfusion is confined to those cases requiring transfusion at very early gestations.

A pre-procedure scan with colour-flow mapping is carried out to establish the site for transfusion. A 20-gauge spinal needle and a needle

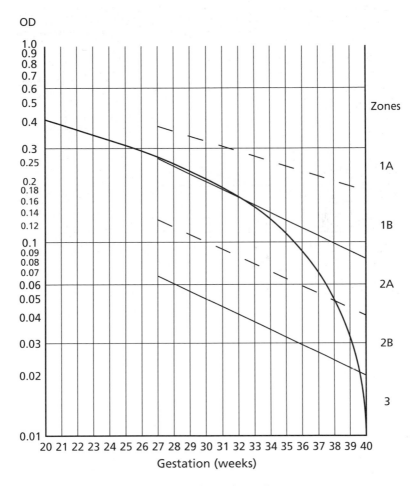

Figure 5.5 Levels of Delta OD450 plotted on Liley curve

guide are used to gain access to the desired vessel (Figure 5.7a: Plate 3). In general, the umbilical vein at the placental cord insertion is chosen and free loops of cord are avoided to minimise the risk of the needle being dislodged by fetal activity. The cord root is most accessible if the placenta is anterior. Posterior placental locations can be more difficult to reach. It may be necessary to give the transfusion via the intrahepatic portion of the umbilical vein but this is dependent on fetal position. Rarely, the transfusion is given via the left ventricle. Occasionally it is necessary to paralyse the fetus with vecuronium 0.25 mg/kg.

With the needle in the vessel a 1–2 ml sample is taken off to check the fetal blood parameters including haematocrit direct Coombs test and

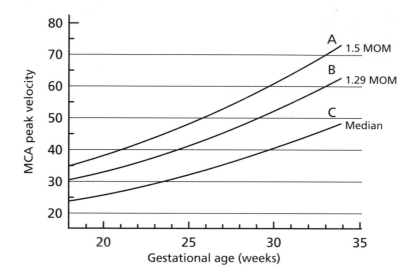

Figure 5.6b Measurement of cerebral artery peak systolic velocity
A = moderate to severe anaemia; B = mild anaemia; C = no anaemia;
MCA = middle cerebral artery; MOM = multiples of the median

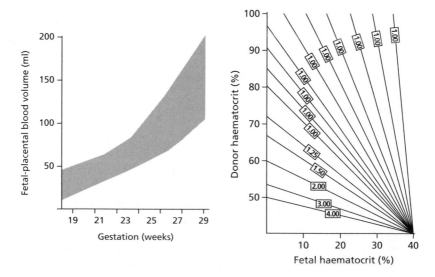

Figure 5.8 Graphs used to calculate volume of blood to be transfused:
(a) fetal placental blood volume: (b) fetal haematocrit

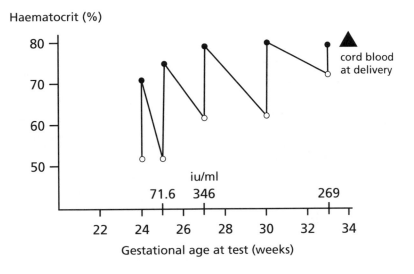

Figure 5.9 Timing of transfusions until delivery

karyotype. A dedicated laboratory team is required for the transfusion procedure; 2 ml of normal saline is flushed through the needle to establish flow in the vessel and the transfusion is commenced while the fetal haematocrit is being measured. O-negative, irradiated, CMV-negative packed red cells are transfused. A donor haematocrit in the region of 70% is preferable as this reduces the volume of transfusion. The laboratory staff calculate the volume of blood to be transfused using a formula incorporating the fetal haematocrit, the haematocrit of the donor blood and the fetoplacental volume (Figure 5.8). Once the required amount has been transfused, the vessel is flushed with 2 ml normal saline and a post-transfusion haematocrit is checked. If this is in the region of 40–45%, the transfusion is discontinued. The injection of blood into the vessel results in turbulence that can be demonstrated ultrasonically. The fetal heart rate is checked intermittently during the procedure. The patient returns to the ward and cardiotocography is carried out. An ultrasound scan is performed the following day and if a satisfactory haematocrit has been reached transfusions are repeated at fortnightly intervals until 34 weeks of gestation (Figure 5.9). Induction of labour or caesarean section is organised soon thereafter.

Emergency delivery by caesarean section is sometimes required if the fetus sustains a prolonged bradycardia, and therefore the labour ward staff and the neonatal team should always be informed when transfusions are taking place.

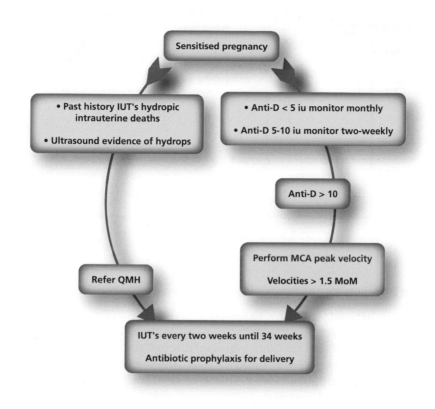

Figure 5.10 Management of rhesus-sensitised pregnancies; algorithm developed for use at the Queen Mother's Hospital, Glasgow (QMH); IUTs = intrauterine transfusions; MCA = middle cerebral artery

An algorithm developed for use in the west of Scotland has been developed and is illustrated in Figure 5.10.

FETOMATERNAL NEONATAL ALLOIMMUNE THROMBOCYTOPENIA

Fetomaternal alloimmune thrombocytopenia (FMAIT) is the platelet equivalent of Rh disease. It is caused by maternal alloimmunisation against a fetal platelet antigen (usually HPA-1 or HPA-2) and the subsequent transfer of maternal antibodies across the placenta into the fetal circulation resulting in a thrombocytopenic fetus. FMAIT is uncommon, occurring at a rate of one in 1000–2000 live births. Infant morbidity and mortality, however, are high, with intracranial haemorrhage being the most severe complication. This occurs in 10–30% of neonates affected by fetal alloimmune thrombocytopenia and is thought to have occurred *in utero* in half of these cases (Bussel *et al.* 1988). Therapy aimed at preventing this complication must therefore be instituted antenatally. What this therapy should be is still debatable, with several invasive and non-invasive treatment options being available.

Maternal therapy in the form of weekly intravenous immunoglobulin at a dose of 1g/kg has been reported as being successful (Mackenzie *et al.* 1999). The direct therapeutic approach requires fetal blood sampling and serial platelet transfusions if the fetal platelet count is less than 50 000. This needs to be repeated every 7–10 days but is a more hazardous procedure than transfusion for Rh disease, due to the risk of exsanguination from the site of blood sampling. It is likely that a combination of both fetal therapies will give the best results, with intravenous immunoglobulin being best for those cases at the milder end of the disease spectrum.

Fetal shunting procedures

FETAL URINARY TRACT OBSTRUCTION

Fetal obstructive uropathies may involve the upper and lower urinary tract. In utero treatment is only considered if there is a bladder obstruction usually as a result of posterior urethral valves (PUV) in a male fetus. Typically this produces an enlarged fetal bladder, bilateral hydronephrosis and decreased amniotic fluid volume (Figure 5.11). In its most severe form a condition known as 'prune belly' syndrome arises (Figure 5.12: Plate 4), with high mortality due to pulmonary hypoplasia. Fetal therapy for PUV involves the insertion of a catheter or shunt into the fetal bladder to drain urine into the amniotic cavity, thus bypassing the obstruction and preventing fetal kidney damage. The early use of double 'pigtail' catheters placed into the fetal bladder met with highly variable success rates. The criteria for intervention were highly variable, and evaluation of the fetus before treatment was minimal in most cases. In 1994, however, an algorithm was introduced for the prenatal evaluation and selection of fetal candidates for prenatal intervention, and this has greatly improved our ability to predict which fetuses might benefit from intervention and those in whom intervention would not improve the clinical outcome (Johnson *et al.* 1994). The three major steps in this evaluation involve obtaining:

- a fetal karyotype
- a detailed sonographic evaluation to rule out other structural anomalies
- serial urine evaluations to determine the extent of the underlying renal damage present.

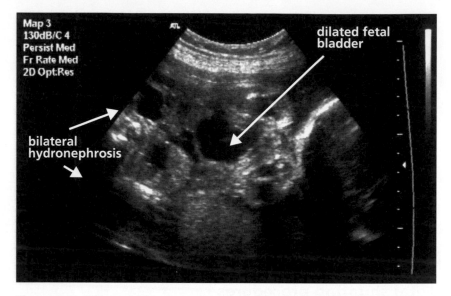

Figure 5.11 Ultrasound appearance of obstructed fetal bladder due to posterior urethral valves

Unfortunately, the predictive ability of ultrasound to identify underlying renal dysplasia accurately is relatively poor. Amnioinfusion using Ringer's solution may be required to both facilitate amniocentesis for karyotyping and to perform a detailed ultrasonic assessment of the fetus. The ranges of biochemical indices in fetal urine at different gestations have been produced from cross-sectional data of individually sampled fetuses with normal renal function, the urine being obtained by fine needle (20-gauge) bladder drainage (vesicocentesis). The importance of serial sampling is well described and must be performed at set intervals for the information to retain its predictive value. It is recommended that the bladder be drained over 48–72 hours and measurements of sodium, chloride, osmolality, calcium, β2-microglobulin and total protein carried out. The urine thresholds for selecting fetuses for intrauterine therapy are shown in Table 5.1. A minimum of three bladder drainages provides optimal predictive value. However, additional drainages may be necessary to establish a clear pattern of decreasing or increasing hypertonicity. The success of intervention for PUV remains controversial. A review of the five largest series reported survival after intervention in 47% and shunt related complications occurred in 45% of cases. Although not all pregnancies had oligohydramnios, of those that did, 56% died despite shunting. Failure to restore amniotic fluid was associated with 100%

Table 5.1	Urine thresholds for selecting fetuses for intrauterine therapy
Sample	Threshold
Sodium	< 100 mg/dl
Chloride	< 90 mg/dl
Osmolality	< 200 mOsm/l
Calcium	< 8 mg/dl
β-2-microglobulin	< 6 mg/dl
Total protein	< 20 mg/dl

mortality. Vesicoamniotic shunting in cases of poor urinary function prognosis was associated with postnatal renal insufficiency in 87.5% of cases and, whereas intervention did improve the chances of survival, it did not alter the renal outcomes. These findings have been illustrated in a follow-up study, which suggested that a significant number of fetuses with so-called good prognostic signs still had a high rate of underlying primary renal dysplasia (Freedman *et al.* 1999).

VESICOAMNIOTIC SHUNTING PROCEDURE

The best results are obtained using the Rodeck-styled double pigtailed shunt. The optimal site for shunt placement is midway between the pubic ramus and the insertion of the umbilical cord. The most common complication is shunt displacement, which often leads to urinary ascites. This can be treated by the insertion of a further shunt to drain the urinary ascites. Shunt placement is performed under simultaneous ultrasound control with the chosen site on the maternal abdomen infiltrated with local anaesthesia. Maternal antibiotic therapy is also administered prior to and following the procedure.

There is agreement among fetal medicine centres performing these invasive procedures that collaborative data should be collected so that the natural history of such conditions and their long-term morbidity and mortality can be accurately defined.

In view of the complications encountered in shunting procedures there has been much interest in the development of alternative therapies. One promising technique is the use of fetal cystoscopic ablation of the posterior valves (Quintero *et al.* 1995). In this procedure, a fetoscope is passed through the shunt cannula and into the proximal urethra until the site of obstruction is visualised. If valves are confirmed, then disruption with a laser is performed. The risks of thin-gauge flexible fetoscopy include amniotic leakage (10%), infection (0.5%) and fetal death (2%). With improvements in instrumentation and experience, this technique may

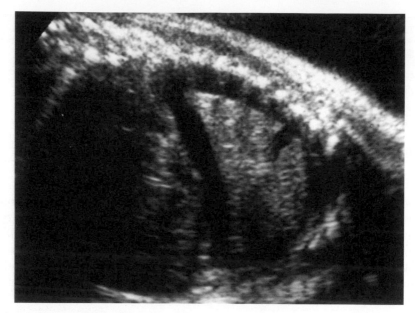

Figure 5.13 Pleural effusion

become the therapy of choice for fetuses with PUV. However, although such techniques are potentially exciting, their use should be subject to strict scrutiny and audit until the natural history of the underlying condition is fully elucidated.

FETAL PLEURAL EFFUSIONS

Fetal pleural effusions occur in approximately one in 10000 pregnancies and may be either primary, usually due to chylothorax, or secondary as a result of aneuploidy or infection(Figure 5.13). They may also lead to NIH. Critical factors determining the eventual neonatal outcome are the aetiology, presence of hydrops, the gestational age at presentation and the ability to offer fetal therapy. As with other potential fetal therapeutic procedures, a detailed search for other anomalies must be made using high-resolution ultrasound and including fetal echocardiography. The couple should have the findings explained and fetal karyotyping should be offered. The overall perinatal mortality is approximately 50% and associated anomalies are found in 40% cases. At the time of karyotyping an aspiration of the pleural fluid can also be performed and this may shed some light on the underlying aetiology. The presence of high mononuclear counts is diagnostic of a chylothorax.

Spontaneous resolution occurs in approximately 10% of cases. If the

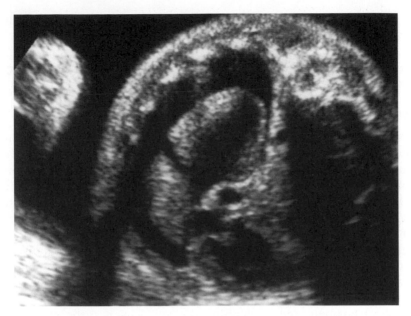

Figure 5.14 Pleural effusion: shunt insertion

effusions are seen before 32 weeks, conservative management is most appropriate if there is no evidence of hydrops and if the effusion is not increasing in severity. In approximately 50% of cases, fetal hydrops is present at the initial presentation or is seen to develop during the time of observation. When hydrops is noted, fetal therapy should be discussed. This consists of thoracentesis and/or placement of a thoracoamniotic shunt (Figures 5.14 and 5.15: Plate 4). The type of shunt used depends on the gestational age of the fetus, the larger Rodeck-style shunts being suitable for the larger fetus, whereas the Somatex shunts are more suitable for the fetus of a lower gestational age. Placement of the shunt is performed under direct ultrasound guidance, using the same technique as is used in bladder shunts. In cases of bilateral effusions, shunts are required on both sides.

In those non-hydropic fetuses treated conservatively, a survival rate of 83% has been reported (Nicolaides 1990). This is in contrast to a survival rate of 12% in hydropic fetuses treated conservatively. Serial thoraco-centeses and thoracoamniotic shunt insertion improve survival especially in the hydropic group. Such fetal therapy may reverse fetal hydrops and polyhydramnios thus reducing the risk of preterm delivery. The extent to which it improves lung development and prevents pulmonary hypoplasia is unknown. Again, few long-term follow up data are available in terms of neonatal/childhood survival and morbidity and prospective evaluation is required. This may involve the use of X-ray and newer imaging techniques such as MRI.

Procedures used to alter the amount of amniotic fluid

AMNIOINFUSION

This technique has been used both as a diagnostic and therapeutic procedure. Often, it is difficult to be clear whether the patient has undergone preterm prelabour rupture of the membranes (PPROM) or if the oligohydramnios is a primary fetal or placental aetiology.

Despite these pathophysiological uncertainties, pregnancies complicated by oligohydramnios at an early gestational age have a poor prognosis due to the strong chance of pulmonary hypoplasia developing. If there is a calculated high probability of associated pulmonary hypoplasia, termination of pregnancy should be discussed. However, it is well known that ultrasound predictors of pulmonary hypoplasia are extremely poor and this is further complicated by the fact that obtaining good views of the fetal anatomy and establishing the aetiology is made even more difficult due to the absence of amniotic fluid which provides the normal acoustic window.

Transabdominal instillation of artificial amniotic fluid is a useful technique used to improve the ultrasound image (Fisk *et al.* 1991). Ringer's solution is usually used with approximately 100–200 ml being infused depending on the gestational age. The procedure is undertaken under simultaneous ultrasound guidance using a 20-gauge needle and a three-way tap. Continuous turbulence of the instilled fluid should be visualised.

The procedure may unmask pre-existing PPROM and this can influence the counselling given to the prospective parents. It is unclear whether repeated amnioinfusion can prevent pulmonary hypoplasia and the potential maternal complications of acute infection must not be underestimated.

AMNIODRAINAGE

This procedure is performed when there is clinical polyhydramnios, which is associated with considerable excess perinatal mortality because of the association between fetal structural anomaly, uteroplacental perfusion abnormality and preterm labour. Medical therapies to reduce liquor volume have included the use of prostaglandin synthetase inhibitors such as indomethacin. The potential adverse effects are both maternal, in terms of gastrointestinal irritation, fluid retention and coagulopathies, and fetal, in terms of premature closure of the ductus arteriosus and cerebral vasoconstriction. The effects are dose-dependent and different dosage regimens are used in the USA (200–400 mg/day) compared with 75–150 mg daily in the UK. The length of time from administration of the drug to it having an effect on amniotic fluid volume is a further disadvantage of medical amnioreduction, since there may be no noticeable clinical effect for seven to ten days. For these reasons, current interest is in the newer cyclo-oxygenase (COX)-2-antagonists such as rofecoxib, since they may be both more effective and have fewer maternal and fetal adverse effects.

Amnioreduction by repeated intermittent amniocentesis can be of benefit in the management of polyhydramnios by reducing intra-amniotic pressure. Repeated amniocenteses do, however, carry an increased risk of infection, preterm delivery and placental abruption.

Amniodrainage is one of the key therapies used in the management of twin-to-twin transfusion syndrome (TTTS). This complication of monochorionic twin pregnancies occurs in 10–15% cases and leads to the development of the oligohydramnios/polyhydramnios sequence. This usually presents at around 20–22 weeks of gestation and can result in a high perinatal mortality (Figure 5.16: Plate 5). The ultrasound diagnosis is based on monochorionicity and the polyhydramnios/oligohydramnios sequence. The sonographic picture includes the presence of a distended fetal bladder in the recipient and the absence of bladder filling in the donor, and, less frequently, discordant fetal sizes. Serial amniodrainages have been the mainstay of therapy for TTTS over the past decade. More recently, fetoscopic laser coagulation of chorionic plate vessels has been introduced. Medical amniotic fluid reduction using maternal administration of indomethacin and digoxin has also been advocated. Amnioreduction has the advantage of being relatively cheap and simple to perform, but there have been concerns regarding the long-term neuro-developmental outcome of the surviving fetuses (Figure 5.17: Plate 5). A retrospective compilation of amniodrainage series published until 1997 and a prospective multicentre study demonstrated a 60% survival rate with about 19% risk for neurological impairment (Ville 1997). The results of laser therapy are discussed later in this chapter. As a result of these studies, a randomised, multicentre trial comparing laser versus amniodrainage in the management of TTTS has been established. Randomisation is carried out online at www.Eurofetus.org.

'Open' fetal surgery

Although most fetal malformations diagnosed antenatally are best managed in the neonatal period, a few severe abnormalities may be better treated by correction before birth. Extensive research using animal models of fetal conditions together with technological advances have led to a growth in human fetal surgery, although at present only a few life-threatening malformations have been successfully corrected. The main obstacles are rupture of the fetal membranes and control of preterm labour.

CONGENITAL DIAPHRAGMATIC HERNIA

The types of fetal malformations that have the potential to be treated by fetal surgery are listed in Table 5.2. The main experience in human fetal cases has been with congenital diaphragmatic hernia (CDH). This condition occurs in one in 2000 to one in 5000 live births. The overall prognosis is dependent upon when and to what extent viscera are herniated into the fetal chest leading to pulmonary hypoplasia (Figure 5.18), as the degree of pulmonary hypoplasia is the most significant determinant of the mortality of CDH, which is 50–60%. The pioneering work in this area has been performed by Michael Harrison and his team in San Francisco. Their initial work involved creating an animal model in fetal lambs and then repairing the defects at various stages of pregnancy. The San Francisco group then extended their work to the human in the form of a clinical trial, which compared fetal surgery with postnatal therapy in a group of fetuses without liver herniation into the fetal chest. Four fetuses diagnosed with CDH underwent correction of the diaphragmatic defect *in utero* and seven fetuses were treated postnatally (Harrison *et al.* 1997). The survival rate was 75% in the fetal group and 86% in the postnatal therapy group. They concluded that fetuses prenatally diagnosed with CDH without liver herniation should be treated postnatally.

A more difficult subset of fetal CDH patients is the group with fetal liver herniated into the chest with associated pulmonary hypoplasia. Ultrasonic

---

Table 5.2   Malformations potentially amenable to fetal surgery

Type of condition	Malformation
Life-threatening	Diaphragmatic hernia
	Cystic adenomatoid malformations
	Posterior urethral valves
	Sacrococcygeal teratoma
	Aqueductal stenosis
	Complete heart block
	Pulmonary artery or aortic obstruction
	Tracheal atresia or stenosis
Non-life-threatening	Myelomeningocele
	Cleft lip and palate

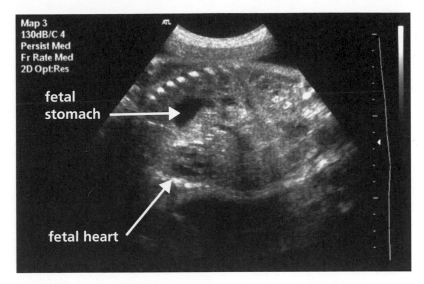

Figure 5.18a Congenital diaphragmatic hernia: longitudinal section through fetal chest and abdomen demonstrating the presence of the fetal stomach and bowel in the chest

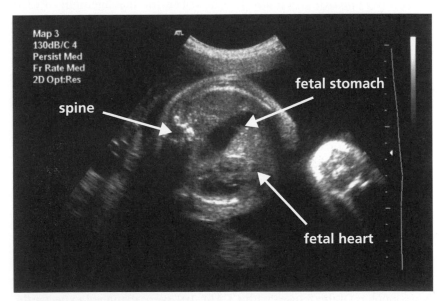

Figure 5.18b Congenital diaphragmatic hernia (CDH): transverse section through the fetal thorax demonstrating a left-sided CDH with the fetal stomach displacing the fetal heart to the right

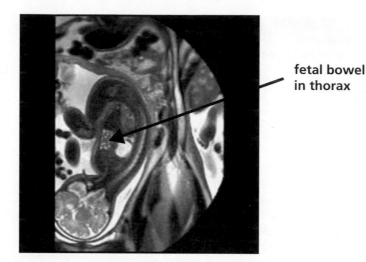

**fetal bowel
in thorax**

Figure 5.19 Fetal MRI showing congenital diaphragmatic hernia

assessment of whether the fetal liver is in the chest is difficult and new imaging techniques such as fetal MRI may prove to be useful in helping to select the most appropriate cases for fetal therapy (Figure 5.19).

The San Francisco group also first described the management of CDH by performing temporary tracheal occlusion, which it is thought enhances fetal lung growth. The initial report was in a group of eight fetuses treated by three different means of tracheal occlusion. The results were poor, with only one long-term survivor, and the technique resulted in variable lung growth. The authors named the technique PLUG: 'plug the lung until it grows' and research in various world centres is currently focusing on the PLUG procedure being performed using minimal access surgical techniques.

FETAL LUNG LESIONS

Two common fetal lung lesions amenable to fetal therapy are congenital cystadenomatoid malformation (CCAM) and bronchopulmonary sequestration. The largest reported series are from Philadelphia and San Francisco (Adzick *et al.* 1998). There were 134 CCAM lesions and 41 bronchopulmonary sequestration lesions over a 15-year period. Broncho-pulmonary sequestration can usually be distinguished from CCAM by the detection of systemic arterial blood supply arising from the aorta on colour flow Doppler. Of the fetuses with CCAM, 101 were managed expectantly, 13 underwent fetal surgery and six had placement of a thoracoamniotic shunt (Figure 5.13). Fetal surgery was carried out in those fetuses with hydrops and solid or multicystic massive lesions. All the fetuses managed conservatively who developed hydrops died before or shortly after birth. Eight of the thirteen hydropic fetuses treated by resection *in utero* between 21 and 29 weeks of gestation survived and continue to do well. The main reason for the poor outcome in the other five cases was preterm labour and development of the maternal 'mirror' syndrome. This occurs when the maternal condition begins to mirror the state of the fetus as was originally described with erythroblastosis fetalis. The maternal signs and symptoms are like pre-eclampsia and include vomiting, hypertension, oedema, proteinuria and pulmonary oedema.

Overall, a dramatic improvement in survival was shown for hydropic fetuses with either *in utero* resection for a massive multicystic or predominantly solid lesion or thoracoamniotic shunting for a single large predominant cyst compared with expectant management.

SACROCOCCYGEAL TERATOMA

The blood supply to a sacrococcygeal teratoma commonly arises from the sacral artery. This vessel can enlarge to the size of the common iliac artery and lead to vascular 'steal' causing high output cardiac failure, placentomegaly, hydrops and ultimately fetal death. If the fetus is mature, caesarean delivery in a tertiary centre adjacent to paediatric surgical facilities should be performed. If hydrops develops prior to 28 weeks of gestation and the teratoma is amenable to resection, then fetal surgery could be considered. A retrospective review of 21 fetal sacrococcygeal teratomas diagnosed over 17 years (1980–97) reported a 19% *in utero* mortality rate and a 14% perinatal mortality rate (Holterman *et al.* 1998). Solid tumours had a particularly poor outcome. Developments in ultrafast fetal MRI (Figure 5.20) may improve the accuracy of antenatal diagnosis and aid counselling.

MYELOMENINGOCELE

Myelomeningocele (spina bifida) is one of the most common fetal malformations in the UK (Figure 4.2: Plate 1). It also has a high rate of prenatal detection due to a combination of maternal serum α-FP screening programmes and because of the reliable cranial signs on routine fetal anomaly scanning.

The rationale for *in utero* repair of neural tube defects arises from experimental work in a fetal lamb model. This work demonstrated that the neurological deficit associated with open neural tube defects is not directly caused by the primary defect but rather is due to chronic mechanical and chemical trauma when the unprotected neural tissue is exposed to the intrauterine environment. Thus, coverage of the

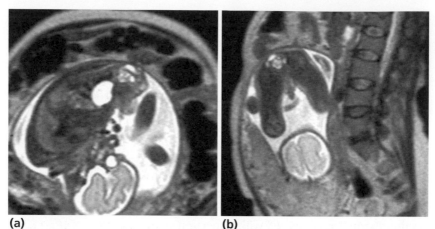

(a)   **(b)**

Figure 5.20 Fetal MRI showing sacrococcygeal teratoma: (a) cross-section;
(b) transverse

myelomeningocele defect with skin flaps could be beneficial and this
procedure has been performed at three centres in the USA. The largest
series is that of the group at Vanderbilt who performed open fetal surgery
on 29 cases of spina bifida (Bruner 1999) and showed that the obstetric
complications are low and the neonatal outcome is improved, particularly
as regards a reduced incidence of ventriculoperitoneal shunting and
almost complete disappearance of the Arnold–Chiari malformation in
those fetuses undergoing fetal surgery compared with a control group
having conventional neonatal care. However, fetal surgery did not appear
to improve bowel or bladder function and is associated with an increased
incidence of premature delivery. It is planned that a multicentre trial will
be conducted in the future.

Minimally invasive fetal surgery

In the 1970s, embryo-fetoscopy was introduced as a merely diagnostic
technique to obtain fetal blood for the diagnosis of haemoglobinopathies
or to directly visualise malformations. The technique was abandoned in
the 1980s because of advances in high-resolution ultrasound imaging.
Developments in endoscopic equipment, especially with the introduction
of small diameter fibrescopes, have increased the technical possibilities
and reduced the invasiveness of endoscopy. Fetoscopy is now also being
used to facilitate operations on the fetus and placenta, and this will
inevitably open up new opportunities to treat the fetus as a patient.

Key elements of the 'new fetoscopy' are the diameter, length field and
angle of vision. Fibre endoscopes with diameters of 1.2–2.3 mm, working

lengths of 25 cm and a 0-degree angle of view are used. The endoscope can be introduced into the amniotic cavity through a sheath. To penetrate the maternal abdomen and uterine wall, the sheath is loaded with a sharp trocar and directed into place using real time ultrasound. The trocar is then withdrawn and the scope is passed. In addition, small instruments such as a laser fibre, forceps or scissors, as well as irrigation, can be used when required. The majority of fetoscopic procedures are performed percutaneously with local anaesthesia and without a formal cannula. However, in complex procedures, such as fetoscopic cord ligation or fetal surgery such as fetoscopic tracheal clipping, multiple cannulae may be required. Such operations may need to be performed through a formal laparotomy.

FETOSCOPIC LASER ABLATION OF PLACENTAL VESSELS

Placental vascular communications exist in virtually all monochorionic pregnancies and only certain vascular patterns lead to the twin-to-twin transfusion syndrome (TTTS). TTTS appears to be based on the presence of one or a few arteriovenous (AV) anastomoses, in combination with a paucity of arterioarterious (AA) or venovenous (VV) anastomoses. The arterioarterious and venovenous anastomoses are found in abundance in uncomplicated monochorionic pregnancies. The arteriovenous anastomosis is not thought to be a true anatomical anastomosis but is considered by some researchers (Van Gemert *et al.* 1998) to be a cotyledon fed by an artery from one fetus and drained by a vein from the other twin. The afferent and efferent branches of this shared cotyledon run over the placental surface and plunge into the chorionic plate almost at the same point. It is thought by some groups that identifying and ablating these vessels results in the elimination of the shared circulation and therefore in the resolution of the abnormal inter-twin blood transfer.

Neodymium:yttrium-aluminium-garnett (Nd:YAG) laser coagulation is usually performed under local or epidural anaesthesia with the use of a percutaneously inserted fetoscope. A 400–600 μm Nd:YAG laser fibre is introduced through the operative sheath. A combination of fetoscopic laser occlusion of chorioangiopagus vessels and systematic coagulation of all vessels crossing the inter-twin membrane is performed. The procedure also involves an amniodrainage procedure as described previously.

Fetal survival following laser ablation has been consistently reported to be around 55–68%, with a risk of about 5% for neurologic injury among survivors (Ville *et al.* 1998). These results appear to have a lower rate of neurological sequelae than the amniodrainage series previously referred to. In a prospective comparative study from Germany, the results of laser ($n = 73$) at one institution were compared prospectively with those of amniodrainage ($n = 43$) at another centre (Hecher *et al.* 1999). The survival rate and neurological morbidity for the laser group were 61% and 6%, respectively, and those for amniodrainage were 51% and 19%. Although this study represents the best comparative data of the two fetal therapies, it suffers from being non-randomised; hence the need for the Eurofetus randomised study discussed previously (www.Eurofetus.org). A multicentre study in the USA is also planned.

FETOSCOPIC CORD OCCLUSION IN COMPLICATED MONOCHORIONIC TWINS

Fetoscopy has been used to assist selective termination by cord occlusion in cases of discordant monochorionic twins. The typical situation is that of the 'twin reversed arterial perfusion' (TRAP) sequence. In TRAP, the blood flows from the umbilical artery of the 'pump' twin in a reversed direction and via an arterioarterious anastomosis into the umbilical artery of the acardiac twin. This occurs in approximately 1% of monochorionic twins and can lead to a situation of high-output cardiac failure in the pump twin.

Other complications of monochorionic twins that may be amenable to cord occlusion include the presence of a major anomaly in one twin, particularly of the central nervous system, and other conditions with a poor prognosis. In such circumstances, conventional techniques for fetocide with intracardiac injection of potassium chloride cannot be carried out in view of the shared circulations and hence the likelihood of fetal death of the unaffected co-twin.

Other procedures have been developed to occlude umbilical blood flow to the affected twin instantly and permanently. These techniques include:

- ultrasound-guided sclerosation or embolisation of major fetal vessels using agents such as absolute alcohol, thrombogenic coils or embucrilate gel (Denbow *et al.* 1998)
- Nd:YAG laser for cord coagulation
- surgical ligation of the cord under either fetoscopic or ultrasound guidance (Deprest *et al.* 1998)
- bipolar coagulation of the umbilical cord under ultrasound guidance (Deprest *et al.* 1998)
- monopolar thermocoagulation under ultrasound guidance (Rodeck *et al.* 1998; Holmes *et al.* 2001).

The success rate for absolute alcohol or enbucrilate gel instillation is only 30% and this technique should therefore now be discouraged. The problem with surgical cord ligation either under fetoscopic or ultrasound guidance is that there is a relatively high rate of PPROM (30%). The preferred procedure for cord ablation is either mono or bipolar coagulation under ultrasound guidance and this technique can be performed in most fetal medicine units.

LYSIS OF AMNIOTIC BANDS

Amniotic band syndrome is a sporadic condition that occurs in approximately one in 1200 to one in 15 000 live births. It can result in serious fetal deformities such as amputations and constrictions. If the diagnosis is made by ultrasound early then fetal therapy can be administered in the form of lysis of the bands using fetoscopic techniques (Quintero *et al.* 1997).

COMPLICATIONS OF OPERATIVE FETOSCOPY

The most important adverse effect of operative fetoscopy is the high risk of PPROM. Even after the 'learning curve' of the procedure, the incidence of iatrogenic PPROM remains significant. Other complications are the same as those with serial amnioreductions such as chorioamnionitis and placental abruption. Since the 'new fetoscopy' is a new method of fetal therapy, it is vital that prospective audit of the fetoscopic techniques performed in fetal medicine centres takes place. A registry of such fetoscopic procedures performed worldwide has now been established whose primary objective is to establish accurate data on maternal and fetal safety that can be used in counselling prospective parents (www.Eurofetus.org).

Fetal pain and awareness

In light of the current availability of fetal treatment options there has been considerable ethical and scientific debate concerning fetal pain and awareness. This resulted in the RCOG asking a working party to make

---

IN UTERO STEM CELL TRANSPLANTATION VERSUS POSTNATAL THERAPY

In utero treatment – advantages

- Fetus is pre immune
- Fetus maintains stable long-term chimerism
- Fetus at 16 weeks does not need immunosuppression

Postnatal treatment – disadvantages

- Donor availability
- Graft rejection
- Graft-versus-host disease
- Patient deterioration prior to treatment

---

recommendations (RCOG 1997). They concluded that there is some evidence of fetal awareness above 22 weeks of gestation and have recommended that should invasive fetal procedures be performed at this gestation or above then they should be carried out only after maternal and/or fetal analgesia is administered. This can be given in the form of maternal sedation with opiates prior to the procedure and in some cases the intravascular administration of analgesics such as fentanyl.

Future therapies

STEM CELL TRANSPLANTATION

Bone marrow transplantation can be used to treat many severe congenital and acquired haematological disorders. However, a large number of patients have no compatible donors and this can lead to rejection in the form of graft-versus-host disease, which is induced by T lymphocytes. In view of the natural lack of T cells during early development, fetal liver stem cells can reconstitute the haematopoietic and lymphopoietic systems without producing graft-versus-host disease. In view of this, stem cell transplantation *in utero* has been successfully performed using fetal liver cells during early human fetal development following prenatal diagnosis.

The main indications for fetal stem cell transplantation are:

- chronic granulomatous disease
- severe combined immunodeficiency
- β-thalassaemia
- sickle cell disease
- fetus that will have neonatal organ failure and can be made immune tolerant.

In utero transplantation has been successfully performed in a handful of cases in specialised centres and may offer a promising potential new fetal therapy for the severely sick fetus (Table 5.3).

Table 5.3	World experience of human stem cell therapy				
Year	Centre	Disorder	Source	Gestation (weeks)	Outcome
1986	London	Rhesus disease	Maternal	17	No chimerism
1989	Lyon	Immunodeficiency	Fetal	30	Engraftment
1989	Lyon	Haemoglobinopathy	Fetal	14	Engraftment
1996	Brescia	Immunodeficiency	Paternal	21	Engraftment
1996	Philadelphia	Immunodeficiency	Paternal	16	Engraftment
1996	Stockholm	Haemoglobinopathy	Fetal	13	No chimerism

GENE THERAPY

As the Human Genome Project attempts to map the estimated 50 000–200 000 genes, much is already known regarding the structure of many genes and the mutations which cause disease states. The ultimate goal is to progress from this knowledge to attempting to cure genetic disease by gene therapy. The main areas of research involve identifying the best approaches for gene transfer and whether these should be using physical methods such as direct DNA injection, by liposome fusion or by biological vectors using retro or adenoviruses. Some of the selected disease models that are currently being studied are:

- defects in haematopoietic cell function
- haemophilia
- familial hypercholesterolaemia
- growth deficiency
- cancer
- cystic fibrosis
- muscle gene therapy.

The major issues that remain unresolved are the length of time for which interventions will provide the desired therapeutic effect and whether expression of the transferred gene will really give clinical benefit. As well as aiding in the treatment of genetic diseases, it is likely that gene therapy will have benefit for other conditions that lead to morbidity and in which transfection (the process of infecting cells with purified DNA or RNA isolated from a virus after a specific pretreatment) of the fetus is more efficient than postnatal therapy.

Ethics of fetal therapy

The pregnant woman is under no obligation to confer the status of being a patient on her previable fetus simply because there exists a fetal therapy. The same is true for fetal therapy on the viable fetus, who is properly judged to be a patient. Fetal therapy should be considered when that intervention would benefit the fetus and the risks of the treatment are acceptable to the pregnant woman. McCullough and Chervenak (1994) consider that three criteria should be satisfied:

- when invasive therapy of the viable fetus is reliably judged to have a very high probability of being life saving or of preventing serious or irreversible disease, injury, or handicap for the fetus and for the child that the fetus can become
- when such therapy is reliably judged to involve low mortality risk and low or manageable risk of serious disease, injury or handicap to the viable fetus and the child it can become

- when the mortality risk to the pregnant woman is reliably judged to be very low, and when the risk of disease, injury or handicap to the pregnant woman is reliably judged to be low or manageable.

Such decision making is complex but the obligations owed to the pregnant woman and to the fetal patient as outlined are mandatory and, as this new branch of perinatal medicine grows, it will be essential to apply such ethical considerations to many more areas of fetal therapy.

References

Adzick NS, Harrison MR, Crombleholme TM, Flake AW, Howell LJ. (1998) Fetal lung lesions: management and outcome. *Am J Obstet Gynecol* **179**:884–9.

Blanch G, Walkinshaw SA, Walsh K. (1994) Cardioversion of fetal tachyarrythmias with adenosine. *Lancet* **344**:1646.

Bruner JP, Tulipan N, Paschall RL, Boehm FH, Walsh WF, Silva SR, *et al.* (1999) Fetal surgery for myelomeningocoele and the incidence of shunt dependent hydrocephalus. *JAMA* **282**:1819–25.

Bussel JB, Neonatal Immune Thrombocytopenia Study Group. (1988) Neonatal alloimmune thrombocytopenia (NAIT): information derived from a prospective international registry. *Paediatr Res* **23**:337.

Copel JA, Buyon JP, Kleinman CS. (1994) Successful *in utero* treatment of fetal heart block. *Am J Obstet Gynecol* **173**:1384–90.

Denbow ML, Overton TG, Duncan KR, Cox PM, Fisk NM. (1999) High failure rate of umbilical vessel occlusion by ultrasound guided injection of absolute alcohol or enbucrilate gel. *Prenat Diagn* **19**:527–32.

Deprest JA, Van Ballaer PP, Evrard VA, Peers KH, Spitz B, Steegers EA, *et al.* (1998) Experience with fetoscopic cord ligation. *Eur J Obstet Gynecol Reprod Biol* **81**:157–64.

Deprest JA, Audibert F, Van Schoubroeck D, Hecher K, Mahieu-Caputo D. (2000) Bipolar cord coagulation of the umbilical cord in complicated monochorionic twin pregnancy. *Am J Obstet Gynecol* **182**:340–5.

Fisk NM, Ronderos-Dumit D, Soliani A, Nicolini U, Vaughan J, Rodeck CH. (1991) Diagnostic and therapeutic transabdominal amnioinfusion in oligohydramnios. *Obstet Gynecol* **78**:270–8.

Forest MG, David M. (1992) [Prevention of sexual ambiguity in children with 21-hydroxylase deficiency by treatment *in utero*.] *Pediatrie* **47**;351–7. In French.

Freedman AL, Johnson MP, Smith CA, Gonzalez R, Evans MI. (1999) Long-term outcome in children after antenatal intervention for obstructive uropathies. *Lancet* **354**:374–7.

Harrison MR, Adzick NS, Bullard KM, Farrell JA, Howell LJ, Rosen MA, *et al.* (1997) Correction of congenital diaphragmatic hernia *in utero*. VII: a prospective trial. *J Paediatr Surg* **32**:1637–42.

Hecher K, Plath H, Bregenzer T, Hansmann M, Hackeloer BJ. (1999) Endoscopic laser surgery compared to serial amniocentesis in the treatment of severe twin-twin transfusion. *Am J Obstet Gynecol* **180**:717–24.

Holmes A, Jauniaux E, Rodeck C. (2001) Monopolar thermocoagulation in acardiac twinning. *BJOG* **108**:1000–2.

Holterman AX, Filiatrault D, Lallier M, Youssef S. (1998) The natural history of sacrococcygeal teratomas diagnosed through routine obstetric sonogram: a single institution experience. *J Paediatr Surg* **33**:899–903.

Johnson MP, Bukowski TP, Reitleman C, Isada NB, Pryde PG, Evans MI. (1994) In utero surgical treatment of fetal obstructive uropathy: a new comprehensive approach to identify appropriate candidates for vesicoamniotic shunt therapy. *Am J Obstet Gynecol* **170**:1770–9.

Little J, Ellwood M. (1992) Geographical variation. In: Ellwood JM, Little J, Ellwood JH. *The Epidemiology and Control of Neural Tube Defects.* Oxford: Oxford University Press. p. 96–145.

McCullough LB, Chervenak FA. (1994) *Ethics in Obstetrics and Gynaecology.* New York: Oxford University Press.

Mackenzie FM, Brennand J, Peterkin M, Cameron AD. (1999) Management of fetal alloimmune thrombocytopenia – a less invasive option? *J Obstet Gynecol* **19**;119–21.

Medical Research Council Vitamin Study Research Group. (1991) Prevention of neural tube defects: results of the Medical Research Council Vitamin Study Research Group. *Lancet* **338**:131–7.

Nicolaides KH, Azar GB. Thoraco-amniotic shunting. *Fetal Diagn Ther* 1990;**5**:153–64.

Quintero RA, Hume R, Smith C, Johnson MP, Cotton DB, Romero R, *et al.* (1995) Percutaneous fetal cystoscopy, and endoscopic fulguration of posterior urethral valves. *Am J Obstet Gynecol* **172**:206–9.

Quintero RA, Morales WJ, Phillips J, Kalter CS, Angel JL. (1997) In utero lysis of amniotic bands. *Ultrasound Obstet Gynecol* **10**:316–20.

Rodeck C, Deans A, Jauniaux E. (1998) Thermocoagulation for the early treatment of pregnancy with an acardiac twin. *N Engl J Med* **339**:1293–5.

Royal College of Obstetricians and Gynaecologists. (1999) *Alcohol Consumption in Pregnancy. Guideline No. 9.* London: RCOG Press.

Royal College of Obstetricians and Gynaecologists. (1997) *Fetal Awareness. Report of a working Party.* London: RCOG Press.

Simpson JM, Sharland GK. (1998) Fetal tachycardias: management and outcome of 127 consecutive cases. *Heart* **79**:576–81.

Simpson JM. (2000) Fetal arrythmias. In: Allan L, Hornberger L, Sharland G, editors. *Textbook of Fetal Cardiology.* London: Greenwich Medical Media. p. 421–7.

Van Gemert MJ, Major AL, Scherjon SA. (1998) Placental anatomy, fetal demise and therapeutic intervention in monochorionic twins and the transfusion syndrome: new hypothesis. *Eur J Obstet Gynecol* **78**:53–62.

Ville Y. (1997) Monochorionic twins: 'les liaisons dangereuses'. *Ultrasound Obstet Gynecol* **10**:82–5.

Ville Y, Hecher K, Gagnon A, Sebire N, Hyett J, Nicolaides K. (1998) Endoscopic laser coagulation in the management of severe twin transfusion syndrome. *BJOG* **105**:446–53.

6 Prenatal diagnosis and management of non-immune hydrops fetalis

Introduction

Fetal non-immune hydrops (NIH) is an uncommon but important condition accounting for a disproportionate 3% of overall perinatal mortality (Figure 6.1: Plate 6). With the decline in rhesus isoimmunisation, non-immunological causes have become responsible for the majority of fetal hydrops. With the increasing use of ultrasound, prenatal diagnosis is possible at an earlier gestational age. The variety of conditions that cause or are associated with fetal hydrops makes it a challenge for the obstetrician to find the cause and decide on the management of this pregnancy complication in order to reduce the high perinatal loss.

NIH is defined as generalised oedema of soft tissues irrespective of the presence of effusions or placental oedema without evidence of isoimmunisation (Figures 6.2, 6.3). It is reported to occur in between one in 1500 and one in 4000 pregnancies. However, recent series (Swain *et al.* 1999) would suggest that the current incidence might be as high as one in 800 pregnancies.

It is important to develop a logical sequence for the investigation and obstetric management of NIH. It is recommended to proceed from the least invasive evaluation methods (serum studies, ultrasound, echocardiography) to the more invasive and sophisticated methods (chorionic villus sampling and cordocentesis) and hence it is likely that referral to a fetal medicine department will be required (Table 6.1).

NIH represents an 'end-stage condition' of different disease processes. To improve survival, early diagnosis must be made prenatally. Ultrasound is the single most useful tool not only in the prenatal diagnostic evaluation but also in the assessment of the disease progression in a fetus with NIH.

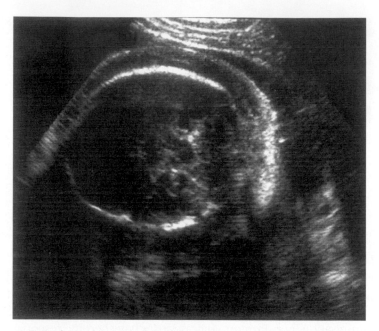

Figure 6.2 Scalp oedema: 'halo' sign

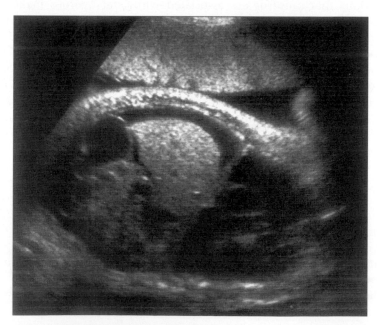

Figure 6.3 Fetal ascites and pleural effusions

Table 6.1   Protocol for the investigation and management of non-immune hydrops (Swain *et al*. 1999)

History
1. Age, parity, gestation
2. Previous scan findings in this pregnancy
3. Past medical and obstetric history
4. Family history (e.g. metabolic disorders)
5. Recent infections and contacts
6. Reason for referral

Maternal investigations
1. Full blood count
2. Blood group and antibodies
3. Haemoglobin electrophoresis (α-thalassaemia carriers)
4. Kleihauer–Betke test (fetomaternal haemorrhage)
5. Infection screening for toxoplasma, cytomegalovirus, rubella, parvovirus, syphilis, serology
6. Autoantibody screen (systemic lupus erythematosus, Anti Ro and La)
7. Oral glucose tolerance test

Fetal investigations
1. Detailed abnormality scan including fetal echocardiography

2. Amniotic fluid index

3. Placental morphology and thickness

4. Doppler flow velocity studies of:
    – umbilical artery
    – middle cerebral artery
    – tricuspid ejection velocity

5. M-mode study of the heart:
    – cardiac biometry
    – heart rate and rhythm

6. Fetal blood sampling:
    – full blood count
    – blood group and Coombs test
    – thalassaemia screen
    – karyotype
    – total IgM
    – glucose-6-phosphate dehydrogenase in male fetuses

7. Viral screen
    – toxoplasma
    – cytomegalovirus
    – rubella virus
    – parvovirus

8. Drainage procedures (fluid aspirated sent for biochemistry and viral screen):
    – pleural effusion
    – ascites
    – amniotic fluid

Aetiology

The major causes are chromosomal abnormality, structural cardiovascular disease, cardiac dysrhythmias, abnormalities of the fetal thorax, haematological disorders and infections. A cause is established in more than half of cases, with no explanation being found in 13–35% of cases. There is an inverse relationship between the incidence of karyotype abnormalities and gestation at presentation and it is unusual not to find a cause in early NIH.

Specific causes

CHROMOSOMAL ABNORMALITIES

Studies from Australia have shown that 52% of cases prior to 20 weeks of gestation have a karyotypic anomaly, whereas 28% of NIH at gestations over 20 weeks have a chromosomal abnormality. The most frequently found abnormalities are trisomy 21 and Turner syndrome, although trisomies 13, 16, 18 and triploidy are not infrequent.

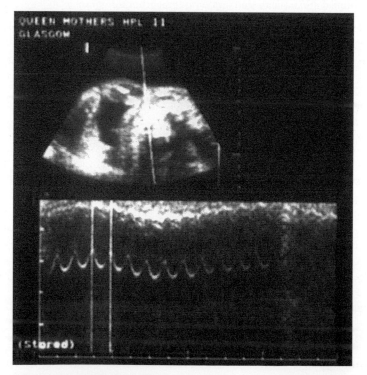

Figure 6.4 Fetal supraventricular tachycardia

CARDIOVASCULAR DISEASE

The combination of anatomical cardiac disease and fetal dysrhythmias makes cardiovascular disease the second most common group of causes. Many of the structural defects also have karyotypic abnormality. Anomalies that lead to increased right-sided atrial pressure are the likeliest to lead to NIH. The lesions with significant left-sided obstruction are the most common, as they result in increased right ventricular flow. Premature closure of the foramen ovale or ductus arteriosus and Ebstein's anomaly also lead to NIH. Hydrops has also been found with septal defects, transposition of the great arteries Fallot's tetralogy and truncus arteriosus.

Fetal cardiac dysrhythmias in the form of either tachy- or bradycardias can also lead to NIH. Tachydysrhythmias are the most common, with supraventricular tachycardia being the cause of 50% of cases (Figure 6.4). Atrioventricular re-entrant tachycardias are the next most frequent and this is followed by atrial flutter. Fetal bradycardias, including congenital complete fetal heart block, are also associated with NIH. These may be associated with either structural congenital heart disease or with maternal connective disorder.

Fetal echocardiography may be indicated if a major cardiac defect is suspected. Recognition of fetal cardiac arrhythmias in the absence of structural cardiac defect offers the opportunity for therapeutic intervention in the form of maternal medication combined with continued observation and planned delivery. This is discussed in more detail in Chapter 5.

ABNORMALITIES OF THE FETAL THORAX

Any space occupying lesion in the chest can lead to NIH. The most common causes are congenital cystic adenomatoid malformation of the lung (CCAM), congenital diaphragmatic hernia, pulmonary sequestration and isolated hydrothorax, including chylothorax. The combination of these pathologies with NIH leads to a poor prognosis in a large percentage of cases. This has led fetal medicine specialists and paediatric surgeons to explore fetal treatment options, including open resection of CCAM during fetal life. Drainage procedures using ultrasound-guided techniques have also been performed in CCAM and in cases of hydrothorax with mixed results. This exciting new area is considered in more detail in Chapter 5.

SKELETAL DYSPLASIAS

Approximately 2–5% of cases of NIH are due to skeletal dysplasia, mainly in those syndromes that have associated severe thoracic restriction, such as thanatophoric dwarfism and Jeune syndrome (asphyxiating thoracic dysplasia).

FETAL AKINESIA SYNDROME

These account for a similar proportion of NIH as the skeletal dysplasias. They include Pena–Shokeir syndrome, myotonic dystrophy, Neu Laxova syndrome and arthrogryposis multiplex. Most of these syndromes are lethal in the neonatal period and have an autosomal recessive inheritance apart from myotonic dystrophy, which is autosomal dominant.

GENETIC CAUSES

A large number of genetic diseases can present as NIH. It is estimated that 10–15% of all NIH are due to genetic diseases that can be grouped into metabolic disorders such as the mucopolysaccharidoses and multiple malformation syndromes, such as Noonan and Cornelia de Lange syndromes. These are important diagnoses to establish, since they have a high (one in four) risk of recurrence.

INVESTIGATION OF NON-INFECTIOUS NIH

Investigation should begin with a detailed maternal history, following which is the key investigation, a detailed high resolution ultrasound scan of the pregnancy. Examination of the fetal anatomy, including fetal echocardiography, should be performed by an experienced ultra-sonographer. This may require referral to a fetal medicine centre. If no obvious structural abnormality is seen, the mother should have further counselling and be offered invasive fetal testing. Chorionic villus sampling should be recommended for those patients with diagnosis of NIH in the late first trimester or early second trimester. In some cases, amniocentesis may be preferred since it allows sampling for viral or bacterial culture and metabolic testing. Liquor should be stored for future testing in those cases where the aetiology is unclear. After 18 weeks, fetal blood sampling by cordocentesis is the preferred invasive test. This allows a rapid diagnosis of chromosomal and metabolic disorders and is also helpful in cases of fetal infections since analysis of fetal plasma for specific immunoglobulin M (IgM) can give an indication of intrauterine infection of fetal tissues. Couples should have in-depth counselling and, in particular, it should be explained that the risk of cordocentesis is higher in cases of NIH. In cases where gross fetal fluid collections are present, these should be drained under ultrasound guidance and the specimen sent to the laboratory for lymphocyte count and protein content evaluation (Figure 6.5). Surviving neonates should have extensive investigations, encompassing a multidisciplinary approach involving medical geneticists and paediatric metabolic medicine specialists in an attempt to obtain a diagnosis. In cases of perinatal loss, a full postmortem examination, including histology,

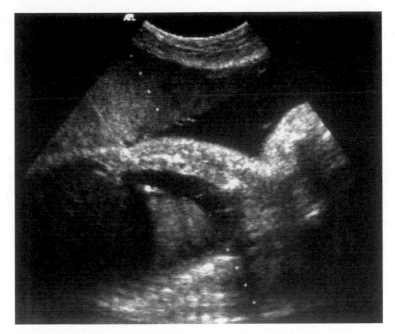

Figure 6.5 Drainage of pleural effusions

should be carried out. In addition, radiology and genetics input may help. Storage of fetal and placental DNA for future studies should go ahead only after full written consent is obtained.

Management of non-infectious NIH

Despite the availability of fetal therapy, for some cases of NIH the overall prognosis for this condition remains poor.

Occasionally, the maternal mirror or Ballantyne syndrome will develop. This leads to severe oedema, proteinuria and hypertension in the mothers of fetuses with NIH, with these symptoms resolving if the fetal hydrops resolves.

In those cases diagnosed early that have such a poor outlook, termination of pregnancy should be discussed. This approach should also be taken when serious associated underlying pathology is also present. The situation of early planned preterm birth should also be avoided since this leads to further morbidity and mortality for the neonate.

Fetal therapy in the form of pleuroamniotic shunting has been successfully attempted in cases where the predominant finding is of pleural effusions but not in the cases of gross fetal ascites with peritoneoamniotic shunting. Other proposed pharmacological treatments have been the use of maternal steroids in cases of complete heart block and digoxin and other antiarrhythmic agents in cardiac dysrhythmias. Some success has also been reported with the use of digoxin and aggressive amnioreduction in cases with non-cardiac cause of NIH.

Fetal infection

Infectious causes contribute approximately 5% of cases with NIH. The specific issues concerning parvovirus are discussed below. Other agents include cytomegalovirus (CMV) and toxoplasmosis. The latter can be treated with maternal therapy using combinations of spiramycin, pyrimethamine and sulfadiazine. Other less common but reported infectious causes of NIH include herpes simplex, listeria and chlamydia. Congenital syphilis can also lead to NIH and this has been successfully treated by maternal high-dose penicillin.

Fetal anaemia

Fetal anaemia is one of the most common causes of NIH, especially if infection by human parvovirus B19 is included. Other haematological causes include α-thalassaemia and glucose-6-phosphate dehydrogenase deficiency. Fetomaternal haemorrhage is also associated with fetal anaemia and NIH. Some of the fetal anaemias, such as those caused by parvovirus, can be treated with intrauterine transfusions.

Human Parvovirus B19 in pregnancy

Parvovirus B19 was discovered in 1975. It is a non-enveloped single-stranded DNA virus, which is the only member of the parvovirus family that is pathogenic in humans, where it replicates in erythroid progenitor cells (Figure 6.6: Plate 6). Parvovirus B19 binds to an antigen in the P-system blood group, which is present on erythrocytes, erythroblasts, megakaryocytes, placental cells, fetal liver and heart cells. Transmission of the virus is via respiratory droplets and the incubation period after contact is one week. This is followed by a period of viraemia lasting approximately four days, with subsequent rash appearing at around 16 days following inoculation. The patient is generally no longer infectious by the time the rash appears. The risk of acquiring parvovirus infection during pregnancy is estimated to be one in 400 and, during an endemic year, there would be two cases of fetal hydrops and 12 spontaneous miscarriages/intrauterine deaths per 100 000 pregnancies. These risks are increased during a parvovirus epidemic. Outbreaks of parvovirus infection show seasonal variation with late winter and spring being the times of peak activity.

Previous infection (IgG positive, IgM negative) probably confers lifelong immunity and it is estimated that approximately 50% of women of childbearing age will show evidence of past infection.

CLINICAL FEATURES

In children parvovirus B19 causes erythema infectiosum, otherwise known as fifth disease. This is a mild influenza-type illness with low-grade pyrexia, which, in some cases, is followed by the development of a characteristic facial rash, known as 'slapped cheek' syndrome (Figure 6.7: Plate 7). In adults, the most common symptom is arthralgia, particularly affecting the hands and knees. Recovery from the infection is usually complete, with no complicating anaemia. However, an aplastic crisis with severe anaemia may result in patients with certain haematological conditions. At least 20% of the population will be asymptomatic in spite of laboratory evidence of infection.

Maternal serology is the first-line investigation to identify 'at-risk' pregnancies. The presence of B19-specific IgM, with or without B19-specific IgG, is indicative of recent infection. The presence of B19-specific IgG alone indicates past infection and therefore immunity. Parvovirus B19 cannot be grown easily in conventional tissue culture and this has limited the diagnostic tests available. The fetus is unable to produce measurable quantities of antibodies prior to 20 weeks of gestation, thus limiting the role of fetal serology in the diagnosis of *in utero* infection. Diagnosis of fetal infection therefore relies upon direct identification of viral particles by electron microscopy, or of viral DNA by fluorescence *in situ* hybridisation or the polymerase chain reaction (PCR). These techniques can be performed on fetal blood, amniotic or ascitic fluid (Figure 6.6: Plate 6). Tissue histology can be used to identify the characteristic intranuclear inclusion bodies, but these will not be present in at least one-third of cases of B19 infection confirmed by other techniques.

EFFECT ON PREGNANCY

Initial reports suggested that the fetal loss rate associated with maternal parvovirus B19 infection was high but these studies were based on small numbers and the cases were identified as a result of adverse outcome rather than primary infection. Subsequent studies have estimated fetal loss rates ranging from 5% to 16%. Fetal loss was most marked when maternal infection occurred at 9–16 weeks of gestation.

Parvovirus infection in animals is associated with characteristic congenital malformations. However, there is no evidence to date to indicate that parvovirus B19 is teratogenic in human pregnancy. In view of this, maternal infection with B19 is not an indication for termination of pregnancy.

Parvovirus B19 infection is an important cause of fetal hydrops (Figure 6.8: Plate 7) and has been implicated in up to 10% of cases of NIH. During epidemics of B19 infection, which occur every two to three years, the frequency of NIH is increased. There are two mechanisms underlying B19-associated hydrops fetalis. First, severe anaemia leads to cardiac failure. Because of the short half-life of erythrocytes, the major target cell of the virus, and the rapid expansion in red blood cell volume, the fetus is particularly susceptible to severe anaemia. However, in contrast to immune hydrops, hydrops secondary to parvovirus infection may present at a relatively mild degree of anaemia, implying an alternative mechanism in its aetiology. Viral particles have been identified in myocardial tissue and it is proposed that cardiac dysfunction secondary to viral myocarditis contributes to the development of cardiac failure.

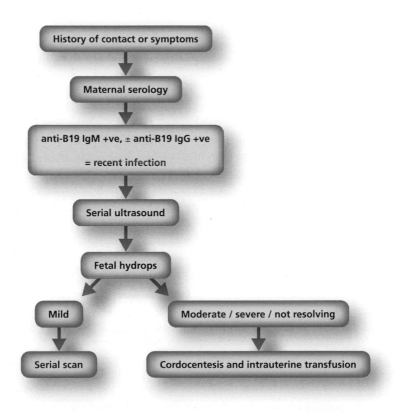

Figure 6.9 Investigation and management of congenital parvovirus infection

MANAGEMENT OF WOMEN INFECTED WITH PARVOVIRUS B19 DURING PREGNANCY

Since NIH secondary to B19 infection is a potentially curable condition, management of a pregnant woman with parvovirus infection is aimed at detecting those fetuses requiring therapeutic intervention. Serial ultrasonography provides the basis for monitoring these pregnancies, looking for signs of hydrops such as scalp oedema, ascites and pericardial/pleural effusions. The placenta often appears large in these cases. Scans are performed at weekly intervals and should be continued for at least eight weeks from the time of exposure.

Continued conservative management may be appropriate for some cases of mild fetal hydrops, since spontaneous resolution can occur, in keeping with the natural history of infection. Failure of the hydrops to resolve or detection of more severe hydrops should prompt a more invasive approach. Intrauterine transfusion has been successfully employed in the treatment of anaemia secondary to parvovirus infection. Cordocentesis is performed to assess the fetal haematocrit and facilities for immediate transfusion should be available. Other tests performed should include karyotype, specific anti-B19 IgG and IgM and detection of viral DNA. A single transfusion is frequently adequate and thereafter noninvasive ultrasound monitoring is essential to ensure resolution. In our own experience there is transient oligohydramnios in the recovery phase following treatment. Cordocentesis is not without risk to the pregnancy and, owing to the fetal condition, the risk is probably higher than that associated with cordocentesis for other indications. A summary of the maternal and fetal investigations and treatment is shown in Figure 6.9 and Table 6.2 (for both see Brennand and Cameron 2000).

POPULATION SCREENING

Fifty percent of adults have serological evidence of past infection and this probably confers lifelong immunity. There will therefore be a percentage

Table 6.2 Laboratory diagnosis of congenital parvovirus infection		
	Sample	*Investigation*
Maternal	Blood	Specific anti-B19 IgM and anti-B 19 IgG
Fetal	Blood or Amniotic fluid or Ascitic fluid	Viral particles (electron microscopy) Viral DNA (FISH or PCR)

of pregnant women who are susceptible to parvovirus B19 and the question is how to reduce this risk. Routine antenatal screening for B19 immunity is not current practice, since there are no measures available that will eliminate the risk of infection. Vaccines are being developed that may dramatically reduce the sequelae of parvovirus in pregnancy, as has been seen with rubella infection, but this remains an area of future research. At present, health education to increase public awareness is important, although the impact that this can make on the rate of parvovirus infection in pregnancy remains limited. Patients with aplastic crisis secondary to parvovirus B19 may be highly contagious and should not be nursed by pregnant healthcare workers. Women who have been in contact with erythema infectiosum should be offered anti-B19 serology to identify those pregnancies that require closer surveillance.

Conclusion

NIH represents a wide spectrum of fetal disease. Many of the aetiologies are associated with an extremely poor outcome. With parvovirus B19 infection, in the majority of cases a successful outcome can be anticipated and, in view of this, parvovirus B19 should be considered in the differential diagnosis of NIH.

The diagnosis, investigation and management of NIH remains both an academic and clinical challenge that should be actively pursued using a multidisciplinary approach in the years ahead.

References

Brennand JE, Cameron AD. (2000) Human parvovirus B19 in pregnancy. *Hosp Med* **61**:93–6.

Swain S, Cameron A, McNay M, Howatson AG. (1999) Prenatal diagnosis and management of nonimmune hydrops fetalis. *Aust N Z J Obstet Gynaecol* **39**:285–90.

Further reading

Cameron AD, Swain S, Patrick WJA. (1997) Human Parvovirus B19 infection associated with Hydrops Fetalis. *Aust N Z J Obstet Gynaecol* **37**:316–19.

Cameron AD, Murphy KW, McNay MB, Mathers AM, Kingdom J, Aitken JA, *et al.* (1994) Midtrimester chorionic villus sampling; an alternative approach? *Am J Obstet Gynecol* **171**:1035–7.

Duthie SJ, Walkinshaw SA. (1995) Parvovirus associated fetal hydrops: reversal of pregnancy induced proteinuric hypertension by *in utero* fetal transfusion. *Br J Obstet Gynaecol* **102**:1011–13.

Jordan JA. (1996) Identification of human parvovirus B19 infection in idiopathic nonimmune hydrops fetalis. *Am J Obstet Gynecol* **174**:37–42.

Kailasam C, Brennand J, Cameron AD. (2001) Congenital parvovirus B19 infection: experience of a recent epidemic. *Fetal Diagn Ther* **16**: 18–22.

Miller E, Fairley CK, Cohen BJ, Seng C. (1998) Immediate and long term outcome of human parvovirus B19 infection in pregnancy. *Br J Obstet Gynaecol* **105**:174–8.

Ryan G, Whittle MJ. (1995) Immune and nonimmune fetal hydrops. In: Reed GB, Claireaux AE, Cockburn F, editors. *Diseases of the Fetus and Newborn,* 2nd ed. London: Chapman and Hall. p. 1257–65.

Walkinshaw SA. (2000) Non-immune fetal hydrops. In: Twining P, McHugo J, Pilling D, editors. *Textbook of Fetal Abnormalities*. WB Saunders. p. 411–26.

7 Termination of pregnancy for fetal abnormality

Introduction

The United Kingdom Abortion Act was passed in 1967 and the Act was amended in 1990 when the Human Fertilisation and Embryology Act was passed. The main changes were that an upper time limit of 24 weeks was introduced for the termination of pregnancy where fetal abnormality was not the indication for the procedure. There was also the removal of any time limit if a termination was being carried out for fetal abnormality, such that no offence was committed under either the law relating to abortion or the Infant Life Preservation Act 1929 if a medical practitioner was involved within the clauses of the Abortion Act in this work.

The main clause concerning termination for fetal abnormality is found in Section I (d) of the Act and this states that termination is permitted when two registered medical practitioners are of an opinion formed in good faith that 'there is substantial risk that if the child were born it would suffer from such physical or mental abnormalities as to be seriously handicapped'.

This, therefore, forms the basis of legal abortion for fetal abnormality in the UK. The stage of pregnancy at which the diagnosis is made, and the time of pregnancy when the decision to perform a termination is made, are crucial in terms of how the procedure may be performed. The decision to terminate a pregnancy because of fetal abnormality is often extremely difficult and it is vital that a comprehensive counselling service is available to the couple concerned prior to undertaking the procedure. This should involve multidisciplinary teamwork from obstetricians, midwives, geneticists and paediatricians, where appropriate.

First trimester of pregnancy

The majority of fetal malformations detected in the first trimester are diagnosed between 10 and 14 weeks of gestation. At this stage of pregnancy the method of choice for termination is vacuum aspiration. Although abortion can be induced by antigestagens and prostaglandins, the incidence of incomplete abortion is high and hence many women require surgical evacuation of the uterus. When performing suction termination, the cervix should be pre-treated using a prostaglandin analogue, such as gemeprost 1 mg vaginally or the prostaglandin E1 analogue misoprostol 400 µg (2 x 200 µg tabs) vaginally. Both these cervical ripening agents need to be administered three hours before surgery for maximal benefit. Although vacuum aspiration is an extremely safe operation, rates of blood loss and other complications rise as gestation advances. Haemorrhage at the time of abortion is rare, complicating around 1.5/1000 abortions overall. The rate is lower for early abortions (1.2/1000 at less than 13 weeks and 8.5/1000 at over 20 weeks). Uterine perforation at the time of surgical abortion is rare. The incidence is approximately 1.4/1000, with the rate being lower early in pregnancy and performed by experienced clinicians. This is also the case as regards cervical trauma, which occurs in less than 1% of cases. Genital tract infection of varying degrees of severity occurs in up to 10% of cases. It is important, therefore, to refer the woman for abortion promptly after the decision to terminate the pregnancy has been made.

Mid-trimester abortion

It is possible to induce abortion at this stage of pregnancy either medically or surgically. Surgical dilatation and evacuation (D&E) is the method of choice in the USA but in the UK its use is confined largely to gynaecologists in private practice. It may be necessary to dilate the cervix up to a diameter of 20 mm before the fetal parts can be extracted. This procedure is associated with long-term morbidity in the form of cervical weakness.

The alternative medical methods involve inducing uterine contractions so that the fetus is expelled from the uterus. In the past, a variety of substances, such as hypertonic saline and urea, together with prostaglandin, were either injected directly into the amniotic sac or instilled through the cervix into the extra-amniotic space using a Foley catheter connected to a pump. These methods were relatively inefficient and labour was prolonged, in some cases for more than 48 hours and, therefore, carried a substantial increase in the risk of infection. There was also the risk of cardiovascular collapse due to inadvertent injection of prostaglandin or hypertonic solution directly into the bloodstream. Instillation has largely been replaced by vaginal prostaglandins in combination with mifepristone pretreatment.

It is well-established that the administration of mifepristone (a progesterone antagonist) 36 to 48 hours prior to induction of abortion with prostaglandins will significantly reduce the induction-to-abortion interval (El-Refaey and Templeton 1995). Therefore, women should be given the option of this treatment. The dose of mifepristone is a single oral dose of 200 mg.

It is the responsibility of the doctor prescribing the mifepristone to make sure that there are no contraindications to treatment. Once administered, the patient should remain in hospital for up to one hour to ensure that there are no adverse effects (occasionally nausea and vomiting). The patient can then go home to be readmitted 36–48 hours later.

On admission, the patient is clerked in and a full blood count, group and save are sent. A cannula should be sited but there is no need to commence intravenous fluids immediately. Abortion is induced with the prostaglandin E1 analogue misoprostol. Alternatively, the other analogue, gemeprost 1 mg, can be given. This is administered vaginally. With misoprostol, the first dose is 800 μg vaginally followed by 400 μg doses orally on a three-hourly basis, to a maximum of five doses in total. For gemeprost, the dose is 1 mg repeated at intervals of three hours, up to a maximum of five doses in total. If a lubricant is required with either of these preparations, a water-based lubricant jelly (such as KY Jelly®, Johnson & Johnson) should be used, not hibitane obstetric cream, as this can inhibit absorption of the prostaglandin. The relative contraindications to prostaglandin treatment are:

- moderate to severe asthma
- allergy or previous hyperstimulation with prostaglandins
- previous uterine surgery.

All patients with previous uterine surgery (e.g. caesarean section) must be discussed with senior medical staff. For such patients, particularly at the ≥ 22 weeks of gestation, the above treatment regimen may need to be altered. Other regimens are described in the RCOG (2000) evidence-based guideline on the care of women requesting induced abortion.

It has been shown, using the above regimen of misoprostol (at gestations of 13–20 weeks) that abortion will be achieved in up to 97% of women. The prostaglandin induction-to-abortion time was six hours and 62% of women aborted following two doses of misoprostol. The women should be fasted after the administration of the first pessary, and

Table 7.1	Dosage of anti-D for rhesus-negative patients
Gestation	*Dose*
< 20 weeks	250 iu
20 weeks	500 iu

intravenous fluids commenced if abortion has not occurred by eight hours after the first pessary.

Most women find the procedure painful and distressing and require opiate analgesia. Normally this should be prescribed as diamorphine 5–10 mg intramuscularly, three-hourly as required for pain. Non-steroidal anti-inflammatory drugs should be avoided.

At the time of the patient's discharge anti-D must be administered if the patient is Rh-negative. The dosage varies according to gestation (Table 7.1). A Kleihauer test should be performed to ensure that the dose given is adequate.

Bromocriptine should be administered from 20 weeks of gestation to suppress lactation, 2.5 mg on the first day, followed by 2.5 mg twice daily for 14 days. The general practitioner must be informed of the patient's discharge. Appropriate follow-up arrangements should be made with the GP, the patient's consultant or the prepregnancy clinic if required.

Late termination of pregnancy for fetal abnormality

Late diagnosis of fetal abnormality may occur as a result of:

- booking late in pregnancy
- an abnormality being missed earlier
- a disorder only diagnosable late in pregnancy; for example, achondroplasia, some forms of genetic microcephaly, severe growth restriction with organ failure, or intracranial haemorrhage such as may occur with alloimmune thrombocytopenia or late viral infection with cytomegalovirus.

Such a diagnosis may lead to psychological harm or mental illness in the mother if she unwillingly continues with the pregnancy, delivers an unwanted child and then has the difficulty of rearing or sending for adoption a baby who is handicapped. The questions raised are whether these interests are grave enough to warrant late termination of pregnancy and whether unwillingness to rear a severely handicapped infant is a morally persuasive reason for termination.

These issues and case examples are found in the RCOG publication on termination of pregnancy for fetal abnormality (RCOG 1996). The recommendations of this and a further working party report on fetal awareness (RCOG 1997) state that if termination is to be carried out after 21 weeks, feticide should be carried out using a technique such as intracardiac injection of potassium chloride, which stops the fetal heart rapidly, with premedication being given to the mother, allowing time for it to build up in the fetus. It is particularly important that there is early discussion with a specialist in fetal medicine both to confirm the diagnosis and to arrange appropriate management. Late feticides should be carried out by trained fetal medicine specialists in recognised fetal medicine centres.

Multifetal pregnancy reduction

Collaborative data from centres with the most experience have shown that multifetal pregnancy reduction can be performed with essentially 100% technical success rate, leading to improved survival and decreased morbidity of fetuses after reduction than there would have been in the high-order multiple births without reduction (Evans *et al.* 1994). Two main techniques have resulted:

- transabdominal needle insertion for injection of intrathoracic potassium chloride
- transvaginal or transcervical aspiration or mechanical disruption of the embryo.

There is no difference in outcome when each procedure has been performed by physicians trained in its use. The transabdominal technique

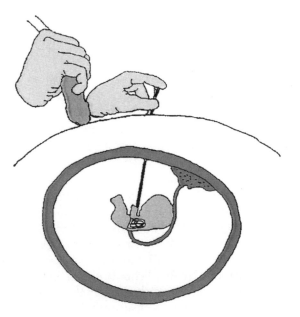

Figure 7.1 Technique used in multifetal pregnancy reduction

requires a thorough ultrasound examination to document proper fetal number and to look for any fetal abnormalities. Measurement of nuchal translucency (NT) in each fetus should also be undertaken, with those fetuses having an increased NT measurement selected for fetal reduction in preference to those with a normal NT measurement. Fetuses demonstrating abnormalities should be selected for reduction but, in practice, it is those fetuses closest to the fundus of the uterus that are easier to reduce. It is also important to look for the appearance of a presumed monozygotic twin pair and these two would be selected for reduction in preference to singletons.

TECHNICAL ASPECTS

The abdomen is washed and draped in the usual manner. Using ultrasound, with or without a biopsy attachment, a spot on the abdomen directly above the sac to be entered is chosen and a 22-gauge needle is inserted through the abdominal wall in a directly vertical approach. Once the needle is in the appropriate sac, it is manoeuvred directly over the thorax of the fetus (Figure 7.1). This insertion must be done briskly since, if pushed slowly, the embryo will merely be pushed out of the way. Once the operator is satisfied that the needle is inside the thorax, the stilette is removed and the syringe with potassium chloride is attached to the end of the needle. The potassium is injected slowly since, if it is inserted too rapidly, this can push the fetus off the tip of the needle. Generally, 0.5–1.0 ml is required to ensure cardiac asystole. The needle should be kept in place to make sure there is no re-initiation of cardiac activity. A new needle is used and the next fetus is then selected in an identical fashion (Figure 7.2).

SELECTIVE TERMINATION

The option of selective termination is available to a mother who has been diagnosed as having one twin with a serious fetal abnormality. Such cases require careful evaluation of the fetal anatomy, followed by a detailed counselling session explaining the underlying diagnosis and the options available. Establishing the diagnosis, providing counselling and performing the techniques should be undertaken in an experienced fetal medicine centre. The first major concern is to ensure that the correct fetus is selected. Although high-resolution ultrasound has made it rare that an abnormal fetus, even one with a chromosomal abnormality, has no detectable morphologic anomalies, occasionally this is still the case. Under these circumstances, it is critical to ensure that the documentation from the laboratory and from the first ultrasound scan under which the amniocentesis or CVS was performed is consistent with what is observed.

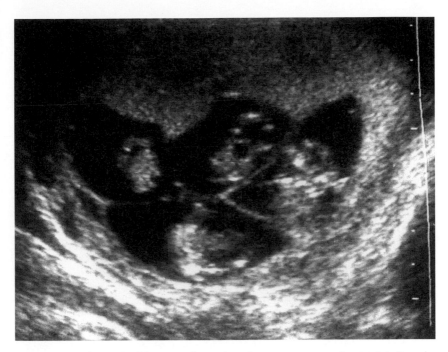

Figure 7.2 Ultrasound image of quadruplet pregnancy prior to fetal reduction

Also, placental position must be observed and a demarcation made between the placentas, to reduce the likelihood of either of the injected potassium chloride or coagulation products affecting the other twin.

A 20-gauge spinal needle is inserted transabdominally directly over the fetal thorax under sterile conditions. The needle should be placed directly into the fetal cardiac chamber and the return of blood seen. Once the needle has been correctly positioned, approximately 2 ml of potassium chloride is injected over 20 seconds. This will usually produce cardiac asystole. However, depending on the gestational age, another 1–7 ml may sometimes be necessary. The needle should not be removed until cardiac asystole is confirmed.

The safety of selective termination depends on lack of vascular communication between the fetuses. The technique described above is not appropriate where there is one placenta with apparent vascular communication between the two fetuses. In such circumstances, a number of other techniques have been used with the best success being obtained with direct fetoscopic ligation of the umbilical cord of the affected twin. Even more recently (Deprest *et al.* 1998), diathermy ablation of the cord has been attempted under direct ultrasound vision.

The collaborative data suggest that a selective termination can be done safely and effectively with an overall fetal loss rate of approximately 5% when the procedure is done at less than 17 weeks of gestation and 15% thereafter.

Conclusion

Termination of pregnancy for fetal abnormality is a sensitive and emotive subject that leads to a great deal of moral and ethical debate. The main role of the health professionals involved in this area is to provide accurate non-directive counselling concerning the specific abnormality that has been identified and to provide a supportive role for the couple once their decision has been made. A further role is to organise up-to-date protocols that deliver an efficient and safe method of terminating the pregnancy.

References

Deprest JA, Van Ballaer PD, Evrard VA, Peers KH, Spitz B, Steegers EA, et al. (1998) Experience with fetoscopic cord ligation. *Eur J Obstet Gynecol Reprod Biol* **81**:157–64.

El-Refaey H, Templeton AA. (1995) Induction of abortion in the second trimester by a combination of mifeprostol and mifepristone: a randomized comparison between two misoprostol regimens. *Hum Reprod* **10**:475–8.

Evans MI, Dommergues M, Timor-Tritsch I, Zador IE, Wapner RJ, Lynch L, et al. (1994) Transabdominal versus transcervical and transvaginal multi-fetal pregnancy reduction: international collaborative experience of more than one thousand cases. *Am J Obstet Gynecol* **170**:902–9.

Royal College of Obstetricians and Gynaecologists. (1996) *Termination of Pregnancy for Fetal Abnormality in England, Wales and Scotland*. London: RCOG Press.

Royal College of Obstetricians and Gynaecologists. (1997) *Fetal Awareness: Report of Working Party*. London: RCOG Press.

Royal College of Obstetricians and Gynaecologists. (2000) *The Care of Women Requesting Induced Abortion. Evidence-based Guideline No. 7*. London: RCOG Press.

8 Intrauterine growth restriction

Introduction

Approximately 5–10% of pregnancies result in the delivery of a small neonate. The majority are simply statistically small for their gestational age (SGA), have grown at a constant velocity and are otherwise healthy. A minority are born small as a result of growth restriction *in utero*. This may be due to one of many pathological processes (Table 8.1) but in most cases while there is neonatal evidence of intrauterine starvation – dry wrinkled skin, loss of adipose tissue and muscle wasting – no specific underlying aetiology can be identified. These cases of 'unexplained intrauterine growth restriction' have been attributed to 'uteroplacental insufficiency'.

Normal uteroplacental development

The fertilised ovum undergoes multiple cell divisions to form the blastocyst as it migrates to the uterine cavity. Once there, it adheres to the

Table 8.1 Pathological causes of intrauterine growth restriction

Causes of SGA pregnancies	Pathology
Chromosome anomalies	Triploidy Trisomy 21, 18, 13
Congenital infection	First trimester exposure to rubella Cytomegalovirus Toxoplasmosis
Structural abnormalities	Skeletal dysplasias Dwarfism Gastoschisis
Teratogens	First trimester exposure to warfarin Fetal alcohol syndrome

SGA = small for gestational age

endometrium and the outer layer of cells, the syncytiotrophoblast, invades the endometrial endothelium, implanting the early pregnancy firmly within the endometrial stroma. Implantation is complete by 10–12 days post-fertilisation. In order to facilitate further growth of the pregnancy, the conceptus must establish a more formal link with the maternal circulation, the placenta (Figure 8.1).

During the next eight weeks the syncytiotrophoblast continues to invade the maternal stroma, extending as far as the decidual/myometrial junction, engulfing small maternal vessels on the way. A framework of core placental villi develops, forming the basic placental structure. Vessels are formed within these villi to generate a placental circulation. This first wave of trophoblast invasion into the endometrium, unlike that of malignant tumours, is precisely regulated and is complete by the end of the first trimester.

At around fourteen weeks of gestation, infiltration of the maternal tissues recommences and invasive trophoblast cells penetrate the

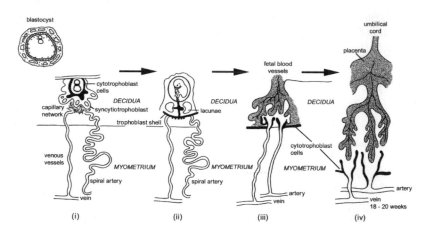

Figure 8.1 Summary of early placental development: (i) and (ii) the blastocyst implants: outer syncytiotrophoblast invades maternal tissues; as the syncytiotrophoblast enlarges, lacunae appear within it; cytotrophoblast cells proliferate and extend to the outer limits of the conceptus forming the trophoblast shell; from this, the formal villous tree will develop by proliferation of the cytotrophoblast and differentiation into syncytiotrophoblast; (iii) the villous stems are vascularised from within to form a formal fetal circulation linking with the umbilical vessel; (iv) the invading cytotrophoblast cells convert the spiral arteries into flaccid vessels and the second wave of trophoblast invasion is complete

myometrial portion of the maternal spiral arteries. The elastic media and muscle of the arteries are destroyed and replaced by fibrinoid material. Without a muscular layer, these resistance vessels become flaccid tubes that easily accommodate increased blood flow to the placental bed. The second wave of trophoblast invasion and modification of the spiral arteries is complete by 18–20 weeks of gestation. Within the placenta itself, multiple small villi grow out from the original core villi, increasing the surface area available for fetomaternal exchange. Because the villous tree contains a rich network of fetal vessels (Figure 8.2: Plate 8), there is rapid transfer of nutrients and waste products to and from the fetus.

Uteroplacental development in IUGR

Uteroplacental blood flow is reduced by more than 50% in pregnancies complicated by IUGR. This is due to a failure of the second wave of trophoblast invasion, resulting in persistence of the muscularised spiral arterial vessels. The underlying cause of this remains unclear. In addition, there is a failure of villous development within the placenta, which severely restricts the surface area available for gas and nutrient exchange. The IUGR fetus therefore not only has a depleted flow of blood into the placental bed but also a limited area for uptake of the available substrates.

Antenatal features of IUGR pregnancies

In the absence of a previous history or significant maternal disease, most pregnancies affected by IUGR present with clinical evidence of a small baby on palpation or reduced fetal movements. Ultrasound-derived measurements of fetal size, employing head circumference, abdominal circumference and femur length, can confirm the small fetus to within 10–15% of the actual birthweight. However, distinguishing the constitutionally small but healthy fetus from one that is pathologically small and at risk is more difficult. Ultrasound parameters (Figure 8.3) such as amniotic fluid volume, umbilical artery Doppler studies and cardiotocography (CTG) can help to assess the fetus. Having identified a growth-restricted baby, Doppler studies of other fetal vessels, such as those in the cerebral circulation, may help to plan timing of delivery.

Cardiotocography

External recording of the fetal heart rate and uterine activity (cardiotocography) has been utilised for almost three decades. A reactive CTG is associated with a good perinatal outcome. In cases of poor placental function, e.g. hypertension or IUGR, fetal heart rate accelerations are reduced and variability diminished. With increasing fetal

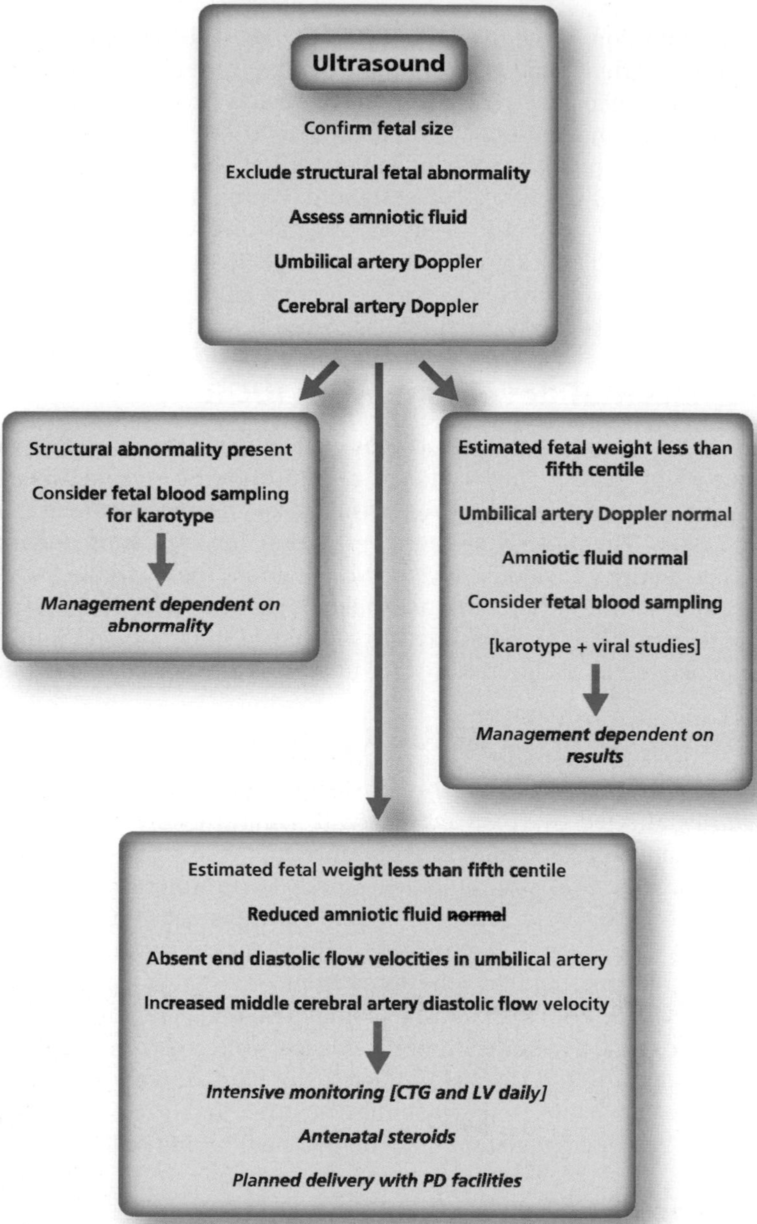

Figure 8.3 The role of ultrasound in the management of a fetus found to be clinically small for gestational age; CTG = cardiotocograph; LV = liquor volume; PD = paediatric department

compromise, variability lessens further and decelerations then appear. These features are related to fetal hypoxia, malnutrition, acidaemia and, in the absence of intervention, fetal death. Where the fetus has reached a viable gestation and is normally formed, delivery by caesarean section, even in the presence of recurrent decelerations, is associated with reasonably good perinatal outcome.

Amniotic fluid volume

During the second half of pregnancy, the fetal kidneys are the main source of amniotic fluid. The amniotic fluid is then swallowed by the fetus, absorbed from the fetal gut into the fetal bloodstream and then circulated through the renal glomeruli to produce more fetal urine. In the absence of premature rupture of the membranes or structural abnormalities in the kidneys, reduced amniotic fluid volumes are thought to reflect impaired renal perfusion. Renal blood flow is reduced if the fetus is hypoxic or hypovolaemic and blood flow is prioritised to vital organs such as the heart and brain at the expense of non-essential organs such as the kidneys. Reduced amniotic fluid volumes are therefore an indirect measure of placental function and fetal hypoxia, particularly in the preterm fetus.

Doppler waveforms

Doppler ultrasound permits non-invasive *in vivo* evaluation of fetal blood flow by using the Doppler principle. This states that a sound wave reflected from a moving target, such as blood cells, will return at a different frequency from the incident sound wave emitted. The change in soundwave frequency, which is proportional to the velocity of the

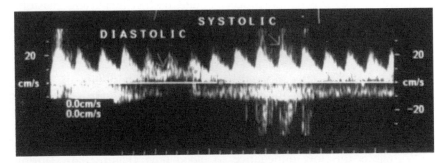

Figure 8.4 Umbilical Doppler studies from the umbilical vein and an umbilical artery; the upper (arterial) waveform changes with the cardiac cycle but even during diastole there is forward flow velocity

moving object, is known as the frequency shift or Doppler shift (Trudinger *et al.* 1985).

In arterial vessels, blood flow is more rapid during systole than in diastole while in veins blood flow is generally constant throughout the cardiac cycle. Within vessels there are also differences. Blood flow in the centre of a vessel is more rapid than blood flow near the vessel wall. At any one point in a vessel, there is therefore a spectrum of frequency shifts, each reflecting different blood flow velocity. Each of these measurements are recorded, averaged by computer and plotted against time to produce a smooth waveform known as the flow velocity waveform (FVW) (Figure 8.4).

A qualitative assessment of blood flow within the fetoplacental circulation may be derived from the diastolic component of the FVW (Figure 8.4). This portion of the FVW reflects downstream impedance within the vessel being examined and is independent of any other variable such as fetal size or blood volume. Several indices have been derived to describe the FVW.

Indices describing the flow velocity waveform

A/B or S/D ratio	=	the ratio of peak systolic (S) to maximal distolic (D) flow velocity
Resistance index (RI)	=	S-D/S
Pulsatility index (PI)	=	S-D/mean velocity

There are standard tables available for the normal range of these indices at different gestational ages. All three indices are highly correlated and fall in value as the pregnancy proceeds, due to the increasing diastolic velocities seen with advancing gestation.

Umbilical artery Doppler studies

Placental vascular impedance falls with advancing gestation in normal pregnancy. This permits the enlarging fetal blood volume to circulate freely through the placenta and ensures that adequate nutritional substrates are extracted from the maternal circulation to supply the growing fetus. The large diastolic component seen in the umbilical artery FVW reflects this low impedance to blood flow (Figure 8.4). During normal pregnancy the RI falls from around 0.9 in the early second trimester to 0.6–0.7 in the third trimester. In pregnancies complicated by severe IUGR, however, the diastolic component of the FVW is reduced,

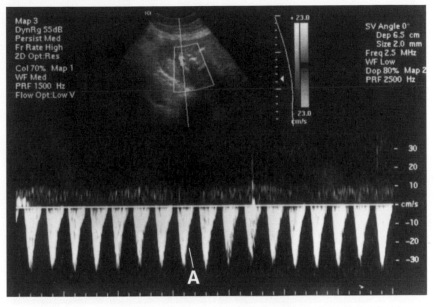

Figure 8.5 The flow velocity waveform is absent during diastole in the umbilical artery (A) waveform from this fetus with severe growth restriction

absent or even reversed (Figure 8.5), indicating increased placental impedance and reduced placental perfusion. As a consequence, there is limited uptake of oxygen and nutrients from the maternal circulation, impairing fetal growth and inducing a 'starvation state'. Perinatal morbidity and mortality are directly correlated with reduced/absent/reversed diastolic flow velocity in the umbilical artery Doppler waveform.

Fetal blood flow distribution in the IUGR fetus

The changes in placental perfusion and substrate supply affect the distribution of blood flow within the fetus. These can be visualised by Doppler studies of specific fetal vessels.

CEREBRAL BLOOD FLOW

During normal pregnancy, impedance to blood flow in the fetal cerebral vessels decreases with advancing gestation, facilitating an increase in blood flow through the cerebral circulation. This is reflected by a fall in middle cerebral resistance measurements from around 28 weeks of gestation. In pregnancies affected by severe IUGR, middle cerebral artery

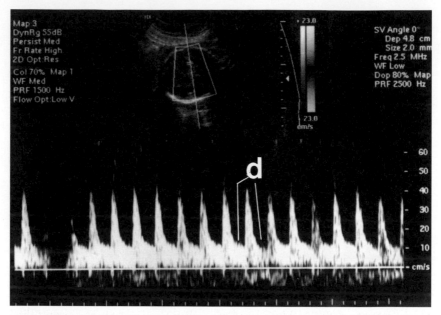

Figure 8.6 The diastolic component (d) of the middle cerebral artery Doppler waveform is increased in a fetus with severe growth restriction reflecting 'brain-sparing'

end-diastolic flow velocities and blood flow are higher than normal, resulting in a low PI (Figure 8.6). This is thought to be a protective mechanism, ensuring that cerebral perfusion is maintained. Animal studies have confirmed that chronic fetal hypoxia, hypercapnia and metabolic acidosis are all associated with increased cerebral blood flow sustained by a fall in cerebral resistance (Vyas *et al.* 1990). As hypoxia progresses, maximal cerebral vasodilatation is reached, preventing any further compensation. Beyond this nadir, further hypoxia results only in severe cerebral vasoconstriction, probably due to cerebral oedema, which is recognised to be a preterminal event.

SYSTEMIC CIRCULATION

Aortic blood flow is significantly depleted in the IUGR fetus and as a result, renal perfusion is diminished and urine output reduced. These adaptations may have long-term effects. Growth-restricted fetuses are particularly susceptible to necrotising enterocolitis, a condition associated with mesenteric hypoxia, and they also often demonstrate impaired renal function in the early neonatal period.

CORONARY BLOOD FLOW

Chronic hypoxia results in thickening of the left-ventricular wall and delayed left-ventricular filling, reflected by umbilical vein 'pulsations' and reversed flow in the ductus venosus. These coronary changes may predispose the IUGR fetus to some of the circulatory problems seen in the early neonatal period and correlate with poor perinatal outcome. To maximise cardiac 'sparing' and protect the myocardium from hypoxic damage, coronary angioneogenesis occurs and increased coronary artery blood flow is facilitated.

Effects of uteroplacental insufficiency on fetal metabolism *in utero*

Data obtained during fetal blood sampling confirm that the growth-restricted fetus with evidence of reduced amniotic fluid and abnormal Doppler studies is hypoxic (Soothill *et al.* 1987), has a metabolic acidosis and shows biochemical evidence of intrauterine starvation (Nicolaides *et al.* 1989) (Table 8.2). As a consequence of hypoxia, erythropoietin levels are increased, stimulating erythroblastosis and macrocytosis, in an effort to improve umbilical vein oxygen content.

Neonatal effects of IUGR

Growth restriction *in utero* predisposes the neonate to complications of low birthweight and, since early delivery is often indicated, prematurity.

Table 8.2   Features of the growth-restricted fetus when compared with a normal fetus *in utero*

Substrate	IUGR fetus
Glucose	Reduced levels
Amino acids	Non-essential to essential amino-acid ratio increased
PO_2	Reduced levels
PCO_2/cord pH	Increased levels/acidotic
Cortisol	Increased concentrations
Lipids	Increased triclycerides
Haematological indices	Erythropoietin increased Platelets reduced Leucocytes reduced

THERMOREGULATION

The growth-restricted neonate has a low ponderal index. Since body length is usually preserved, there is a large surface area available for heat loss. Heat loss is exacerbated by the lack of subcutaneous adipose tissue, a high basal metabolic rate and thin permeable skin.

HYPOGLYCAEMIA

Due to the limited supply of glucose *in utero*, the growth-restricted neonate is born with little adipose tissue and few glycogen reserves. Hypoglycaemia is associated with adverse neurological outcome. To prevent this, early feeding is encouraged and blood glucose levels monitored carefully to ensure adequate caloric intake.

POLYCYTHEMIA

Poor placental function results in chronic fetal hypoxia *in utero*. To maximise oxygen uptake, fetal red-cell production is stimulated and red-cell mass increased. As a consequence, the neonatal haematocrit and blood viscosity is increased. The high red-cell mass increases basal metabolic requirements and also the likelihood of jaundice.

CEREBRAL HAEMORRHAGE

Even minor alterations in cerebral blood flow may have profound effects on the developing brain. Haemorrhage into the parenchyma of the cerebral cortex can result in long-term handicap and/or cerebral palsy, while bleeding into the lateral ventricles may cause occlusion of cerebrospinal fluid and hydrocephalus. Periventricular leucomalacia due to cerebral infarction is less common but more strongly associated with cerebral palsy. The circulatory changes initiated *in utero* predispose the growth-restricted neonate to alterations in cerebral blood flow and these major intracranial events.

CARDIOVASCULAR

Pulmonary hypertension and a persistent fetal circulation are more common in IUGR. Myocardial contractility is often poor and may exacerbate the circulatory problems encountered in the first few weeks of life.

Prediction of IUGR: uterine artery Doppler

Since idiopathic IUGR is due to poor placentation, colour Doppler ultrasound of the uterine arteries has been proposed as a screening test to predict pre-eclampsia and SGA infants. The RI of the uterine arteries is

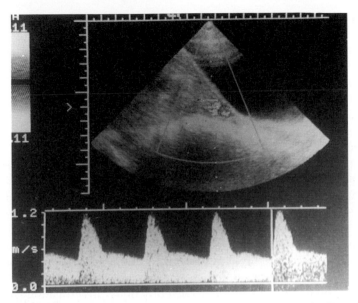

Figure 8.7a A normal uterine artery waveform with a smooth diastolic component

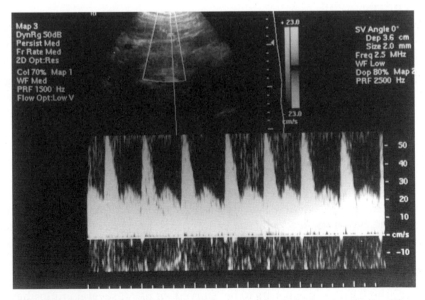

Figure 8.7b The uterine artery waveform at 24 weeks in a patient with a previous pregnancy affected by severe pre-eclampsia; the diastolic notch (n) is still present

used to estimate impedance to blood flow within the uteroplacental circulation. With advancing gestation the RI should fall as the second wave of trophoblast invasion proceeds, converting the muscularised spiral arteries into flaccid vessels (Figure 8.1). When this does not occur and the spiral arteries remain muscularised, impedance within the uteroplacental bed remains high and the RI is elevated. The presence of a 'notch' in the diastolic component of the FVW is also associated with increased impedance, particularly when the notch is bilateral and is still present at 24 weeks (Figures 8.7a and b).

Prospective studies using uterine artery Doppler in the second trimester have been disappointing. While the absence of a diastolic 'notch' and a normal RI are associated with a normal pregnancy outcome, the positive predictive values of this test for growth-restricted fetuses is consistently 25–30%, even when the test is delayed until 22–24 weeks of gestation (Bewley *et al.* 1991; Bower *et al.* 1993; North *et al.* 1994). In order to improve the predictability of uterine artery Doppler studies, the addition of parameters such as maternal serum α-FP levels, maternal blood pressure and platelet function are currently under investigation (Bromley *et al.* 1994; Jaffa *et al.* 1997; Lees *et al.* 1997).

Potential therapies for IUGR

ASPIRIN

Aspirin, in a dosage of 60–150 mg daily, is known to inhibit platelet cyclo-oxygenase and the production of thromboxane, a potent vasoconstrictor. Since the poor uteroplacental blood flow seen in IUGR pregnancies is due to persistence of the vasoactive muscularised spiral arteries, low-dose aspirin has been used as a potential therapy to reduce vasospasm in the uteroplacental circulation and prevent platelet aggregation that may further compromise blood flow.

Once signs of IUGR, such as abnormal umbilical artery Doppler, are present, the introduction of aspirin therapy does not improve clinical outcome. Aspirin may be useful in subsequent pregnancies to reduce the risk of recurrent IUGR. Several studies, including the CLASP trial, have suggested that in women with early-onset IUGR, low-dose aspirin used from the end of the first trimester can improve fetal growth, although the mechanism for this is not clear.

IMPROVED SUBSTRATE SUPPLY

Since the IUGR fetus appears to be 'starved' *in utero*, several groups have attempted to load the maternal circulation with additional substrates in an attempt to improve the available fetal supply. Supplemental oxygen to the mother, which appears to increase fetal arterial oxygen tension in the short term, does not improve oxygen consumption in the fetus in the long term. Furthermore, on cessation of maternal oxygen therapy fetal partial pressure of oxygen (PO_2) falls below pretreatment levels, exacerbating fetal hypoxia further. Glucose and amino acid infusions have likewise proved unsuccessful and in many cases have proved lethal to the fetus.

FUTURE DIRECTIONS

Recent animal work that addresses the primary problem of poor placentation appears to be more promising. Insulin growth factor-1 (IGF-1), is one of many factors that are known to be involved in placental villous and vascular growth. When infused into the maternal circulation of pregnant sheep over several days, not only was placental blood flow improved as demonstrated by umbilical artery Doppler but fetal organ growth also increased (Lok *et al.* 1996). While these animal studies are preliminary, they suggest that by improving primary placenta development, fetal growth and development can also be modified.

Long-term sequelae of restricted fetal growth *in utero*

The effects of IUGR may persist well into adult life. The incidence of hypertension in later life rises as birthweight falls (Barker 1992), and death from cardiovascular disease are strongly correlated with a low ponderal index at birth (Eriksson *et al.* 1999). Serum cholesterol and low-density lipoprotein concentrations, both additional cardiovascular risk factors, are elevated in adults who were low-birthweight babies. Other organs are also affected. The number of renal nephrons is reduced in infants with severe IUGR and the expression of renin-containing cells also increased, both features that may predispose to later hypertension. There appear to be critical periods of organ development during intrauterine life, as yet undefined, which determine later function. Adverse influences, such as nutrient deprivation, during these critical periods may permanently alter the development and physiology of these systems, thus programming the fetus towards adult disease patterns.

Summary

The problem of restricted fetal growth attributed to 'uteroplacental insufficiency' is still poorly understood. Current management is limited to early recognition, close fetal/maternal surveillance and timely delivery in centres with appropriate paediatric facilities.

References

Barker DJP. (1992) *Fetal and Infant Origins of Adult Disease*. London: BMJ Publishing Group. p. 175–86.

Bewley S, Cooper D, Campbell S. (1991) Doppler investigation of uteroplacental blood flow resistance in the second trimester: a screening study for pre-eclampsia and intrauterine growth retardation. *Br J Obstet Gynaecol* **98**:871–9.

Bower S, Schuchter K, Campbell S. (1993) Doppler ultrasound screening as part of routine antenatal scanning: prediction of pre-eclampsia and intrauterine growth retardation. *Br J Obstet Gynaecol* **100**:989–94.

Bromley B, Frigoletto FD, Harlow BL, Pauker S, Benacerraf BR. (1994) The role of Doppler velocimetry in the structurally normal second trimester fetus with elevated levels of maternal serum α-fetoprotein. *Ultrasound Obstet Gynecol* **4**:377–80.

Eriksson JG, Forsen T, Tuomilehto J, Winter PD, Osmond C, Barker DJ. (1999) Catch-up growth in childhood and death from coronary heart disease: longitudinal study. *BMJ* **318**:427–31.

Jaffa A, Yaron Y, Har-Toov J, Amster R, Legum C, Lessing JB. (1997) Doppler velocimetry of the umbilical artery as a predictor of pregnancy outcome in pregnancies characterised by elevated maternal serum alpha-fetoprotein and normal amniotic fluid alpha-fetoprotein. *Fetal Diagn Ther* **12**:85–8.

Lees CC, Brown AS, Harrington KF, Beacon HJ, Martin JF, Campbell S. (1997) A cross-sectional study of platelet volume in normal healthy normotensive women with bilateral uterine artery notches. *Ultrasound Obstet Gynecol* **10**:277–81.

Lok F, Owens JA, Mundy L, Robinson JS, Owens PC. (1996) Insulin-like growth factor 1 promotes growth selectively in fetal sheep in late gestation. *Am J Physiol* **270**:R1148—55.

Nicolaides KH, Economides DL, Soothill PW. (1989) Blood gases, pH, and lactate in appropriate and small-for-gestational-age fetuses. *Am J Obstet Gynecol* **161**:996–1001.

North RA, Ferrier C, Long D, Townend K, Kincaid Smith P. (1994) Uterine artery Doppler flow velocity waveforms in the second trimester for the prediction of pre-eclampsia and fetal growth retardation. *Obstet Gynecol* **83**:378–86.

Soothill P, Nicolaides KH, Campbell S. (1987) Prenatal asphyxia, hyperlacticemia, hypoglycemia and erythroblastosis in growth retarded fetuses. *BMJ* **294**:1051–3.

Trudinger BJ, Giles WB, Cook CM, Bombardien J, Collins L. (1985) Fetal umbilical artery flow velocity waveforms and placental resistance: clinical significance. *Br J Obstet Gynaecol* **92**:23–30.

Vyas S, Nicolaides KH, Bower S, Campbell S. (1990) Middle cerebral artery flow velocity waveforms in fetal hypoxaemia. *Br J Obstet Gynaecol* **97**:797–803.

9 Twin pregnancy

Introduction

The incidence of twin pregnancy has gradually increased over the last decade. In Scotland, twins accounted for 12.7 per 1000 maternities in 1994 and 14.3 per 1000 maternities in 1998 (Registrar General, Scotland). The increase has been attributed in part to the rising number of older mothers, who are at increased risk of multiple pregnancy, and also to the increasing availability of assisted conception techniques. Up to 25–30% of ovulation induction and *in vitro* fertilisation cycles result in a twin pregnancy (Barlow and Mahmud 1995). This presents a significant problem, since despite advances in neonatal medicine both the stillbirth and neonatal death rates in twin pregnancies are up to five times higher than those in singleton pregnancies. Some of the major complications that contribute to these poor perinatal outcomes are discussed in this chapter.

Chorionicity and zygosity

Traditionally, twin pregnancies have been categorised on the basis of zygosity: monozygous or 'identical' twins arising from a single oocyte and dizygous or 'non-identical' twins arising from two separate oocytes. In the

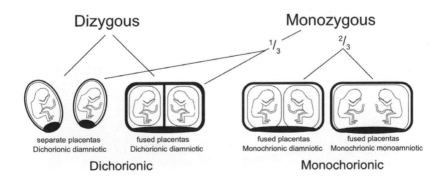

Figure 9.1 The relationship between zygosity and chorionicity

absence of discordant fetal sex, zygosity can only be confirmed postnatally by DNA analysis of fetal or placental tissue. Monozygous twins, having identical genetic material, are ideal subjects for evaluating the effects of environmental or exogenous factors on disease processes. The mechanism for monozygotic twinning is not well understood but the rate is relatively constant, at 3–4 per 1000 maternities throughout the world. Dizygotic twinning is due to an inherited tendency for polyovulation that varies dramatically between different populations. It is this difference in dizygotic twin rates that accounts for the variation in total twin rates worldwide.

Twin pregnancies may also be classified by chorionicity: the number of chorionic membranes present on direct examination of the placenta and membranes following delivery. The terms chorionicity and zygosity are not directly interchangeable (Figure 9.1). While all dizygous twins are dichorionic, only two-thirds of monozygous twins are monochorionic.

PRENATAL DETERMINATION OF CHORIONICITY

With real-time, high-resolution ultrasonography it is now possible to determine chorionicity antenatally. The first trimester (10–14 weeks) is the optimal time to diagnose chorionicity. Where two placental masses are identified on ultrasound examination the pregnancy is dichorionic. More

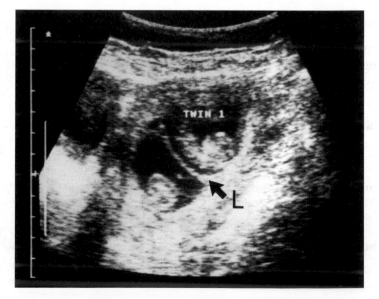

Figure 9.2 The lambda sign; a tongue of placental tissue protrudes into the base of the inter-twin membrane (L)

frequently, a single placental mass exists and chorionicity can only be determined by evaluation of the intertwin membrane. The lambda sign is diagnosed when a tongue of placental tissue protrudes into the base of the inter-twin membrane (Figure 9.2) and this indicates a dichorionic pregnancy. In a monochorionic pregnancy the intertwin membrane inserts directly into the placenta, the T sign (Figure 9.3). With advancing gestational age, these features in the inter-twin membrane are more difficult to identify and by 20 weeks of gestation are only 80% accurate.

During the second trimester, other ultrasound features have been used to determine chorionicity. Discordant genders, the number of placental masses, number of chorionic membranes seen and intertwin membrane thickness have all been evaluated. In expert hands these may be up to 80% accurate, but none have proved as reliable as the first trimester lambda and T sign (Finberg 1992; Sepulveda *et al.* 1996).

IS PRENATAL DETERMINATION OF CHORIONICITY OF VALUE?

With more careful documentation of chorionicity and zygosity during the last decade, it is clear that many complications of twin pregnancies are specific to either monochorionic or dichorionic pregnancies. While

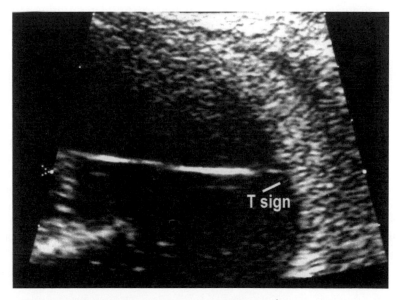

Figure 9.3 The T-sign; the chorionic membrane inserts directly into the placental tissue and indicates a monochorionic twin pregnancy

perinatal mortality is substantially higher in identical twins, chorionicity rather than zygosity appears to be a better determinant of perinatal outcome. Among our series of almost 500 twin pregnancies, the perinatal mortality rate in monochorionic twins was four times that of dichorionic twins. Particular problems in the monochorionic pregnancies, discussed later in this chapter, accounted for most of this difference. Preterm delivery and low birthweight are also seen more commonly in monochorionic pregnancies. In order to target these high-risk cases and tailor care appropriately, chorionicity must be determined. In addition, prenatal testing and the management of an anomalous twin can be planned only if chorionicity is known. Since chorionicity can most accurately be determined in the first trimester, every effort should be made to classify twins before 14 weeks of completed gestation.

Preterm delivery

The median gestation at delivery of a twin pregnancy is only 245 days, with around 25–30% of all twins delivering prior to 37 weeks of completed gestation. While 89% of all twin deaths occur in this group, the vast majority of perinatal deaths (65%) occur in those pregnancies that deliver prior to 28 weeks of gestation. Although some twin complications predispose to premature delivery, unexplained spontaneous preterm labours account for most of the premature births. It has been assumed that uterine overdistension in twin pregnancies stimulates uterine activity and preterm delivery but the pathophysiology of 'spontaneous' preterm labour in twins is not clear.

Predicting preterm labour

FETAL FIBRONECTIN

Fetal fibronectin (FFN) is a glycoprotein present in the extracellular matrix at the uteroplacental interface. It is normally detectable only in cervicovaginal fluids under 20 weeks of gestation and at term. In twin pregnancies, a positive FFN test at 24 or 28 weeks of gestation appears to identify pregnancies at higher risk of preterm delivery, particularly if both samples are positive. However, less than half of all twins who deliver prematurely will have a positive FFN result. These studies need to be validated in larger populations before FFN is introduced more widely as a screening test.

CERVICAL LENGTH

The cervix shortens, softens and dilates ('effacement') with advancing gestation. Digital cervical examination and cervical scoring systems (cervical

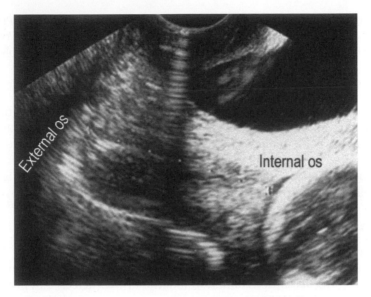

Figure 9.4 Transvaginal ultrasound assessment of the cervical length

length minus cervical dilatation) have been used to predict twin pregnancies at risk of preterm delivery with some success (Neilson *et al.* 1988; Newman *et al.* 1991). Of necessity these systems require a vaginal examination at each visit and are dependent upon consistency between examiners.

Transvaginal ultrasound assessment of the cervix has been evaluated (Figure 9.4). A cervical length of less than 30 mm is thought to indicate increased risk of preterm delivery but in isolation does not appear to be any more sensitive than FFN at predicting delivery less than 32 weeks or less than 35 weeks of gestation. Many of the studies to date have also been complicated by either disclosure of results to clinicians or widespread use of tocolytics.

UTERINE ACTIVITY MONITORING

Women with twin pregnancies frequently present in established preterm labour. While studies have confirmed that uterine activity is present for several hours prior to admission, this is often not appreciated by the patient. Home monitoring of uterine activity in both singleton and multiple pregnancies has been used, primarily in the USA, with some improvement in preterm delivery rates. However, it is difficult to distinguish whether this was a real effect of monitoring or was due to the increased awareness of patients about the signs and symptoms of preterm labour. A meta-analysis of randomised trials on home monitoring demonstrated no significant effect on the rate of preterm delivery in twins but the numbers of twins were small. A more rigorous prospective trial is required before home uterine activity monitoring is dismissed completely.

Treatment of preterm labour

Tocolytics remain the mainstay of treatment once labour is diagnosed. There are no randomised trials that specifically address the use of betamimetics or indomethacin to suppress labour in twin pregnancies. For the moment, the evidence from singleton pregnancies has been extrapolated and tocolytics should be used for 48 hours to suppress labour and allow administration of steroids to promote fetal lung maturity.

Fetal abnormality

The incidence of structural defects is 1.5–2.0 times higher in twins compared with singleton pregnancies. The most common abnormalities seen are CHD, facial clefts, anterior abdominal wall defects and problems affecting the central nervous system, particularly anencephaly. As most of these should be detected by high-resolution sonography, all twin pregnancies should be offered a second-trimester detailed anomaly scan. Structural abnormalities occur more commonly in monochorionic twins, often affecting only one twin. If the abnormality is lethal, most pregnancies will be managed conservatively to allow the unaffected twin to be delivered at around term. When the abnormality is non-lethal but associated with significant handicap, as in spina bifida, some parents may opt to end the entire pregnancy. The options of selective feticide of an affected twin are dependent upon the chorionicity of the pregnancy. Selective feticide in monochorionic twins is associated with a greater than 80% mortality for both twins, since the administration of intracardiac potassium chloride will pass to the co-twin via the placental vascular connections. Umbilical cord ligation of the abnormal twin has also been performed to effect selective feticide (Quintero et al. 1996). No serious adverse morbidity has been reported in surviving co-twins. This technique may well offer a realistic option for the couple who have monochorionic twins with a serious structural abnormality in one fetus. Prior to embarking on any such procedures, the parents should be counselled by specialists in a fetal medicine centre. Selective feticide of an abnormal dichorionic twin may be performed using fetal intracardiac potassium chloride. There is still an associated risk of miscarriage that appears to be gestation-dependent. When feticide is performed at less than 17 weeks of gestation the risk of miscarriage is 5%, but this increases to 15% if feticide is delayed beyond 17 weeks.

Since many twin pregnancies occur in older mothers, chromosome abnormalities such as trisomy 21 are not uncommon. Monochorionic twin pregnancies arise from a single oocyte and will have the same age-related risk of trisomy 21 as a singleton pregnancy in a mother of the same age. A dichorionic twin pregnancy, since it involves two oocytes, will have double the maternal age-related risk of trisomy.

Second-trimester biochemical screening to calculate risks for trisomy 21 in twin pregnancies is fraught with difficulty and is therefore not offered in the majority of maternity units. First-trimester ultrasound measurements of nuchal translucency in twin pregnancies have been reported (Sebire *et al.* 1996). The test appears to be as reliable in dichorionic twins as in a singleton pregnancy, with a low false positive rate. However, in monochorionic twin pregnancies, increased nuchal translucency is more commonly seen, although the karyotype is normal. The false positive rate in monochorionic pregnancies is therefore higher than for singletons. Increased nuchal fluid in a monochorionic twin pregnancy may be due to the shared placental circulations, which results in some twins demonstrating a degree of early cardiovascular failure and dependent nuchal oedema. Despite this, most monochorionic twins with a chromosome abnormality will have an increase in nuchal translucency measurement.

INVASIVE PRENATAL TESTING

Invasive testing in a twin pregnancy necessitates accurate determination of chorionicity and careful documentation of sampling. Monochorionic twin pregnancies require sampling of only one pool of amniotic fluid, placenta or fetus, as the genetic material is identical in both twins. In dichorionic twins both pregnancies must be sampled. Prior to any procedure being performed, the putative parents must be counselled about the possible ethical dilemmas they face if an abnormal karyotype is found in one twin.

Due to the technical difficulties with first-trimester CVS in ensuring that both placentas are sampled, most units offer second-trimester amniocentesis to those parents wishing to have a diagnostic test: most operators use more than one needle insertion to ensure accurate uncontaminated sampling of each sac and, hence, a higher procedure-related fetal loss rate than in singleton pregnancy is to be anticipated (Tabor *et al.* 1986). Centres that perform CVS in twin pregnancies report a loss rate of around 2%, almost the same as that seen in a singleton pregnancy following CVS.

Intrauterine death of one twin

During the first trimester a significant number of twin pregnancies miscarry completely and up to 30% of all pregnancies diagnosed as twins continue as a singleton pregnancy following the demise of one twin. Intrauterine death of one twin in the late second or third trimester occurs in less than

1% of all twin pregnancies but is a difficult dilemma for both parents and obstetricians to deal with. Frequently no specific cause of death can be identified antenatally and even with post-mortem examination, no clear answers may be obtained. In monochorionic pregnancies, the demise of one twin is often a complication of twin-to-twin transfusion syndrome (TTTS), while in dichorionic pregnancies problems such as intrauterine growth restriction with or without pre-eclampsia, fetal abnormality and cord accidents are more common causes of death.

COMPLICATIONS IN THE SURVIVING CO-TWIN

Surviving co-twins in both monochorionic and dichorionic pregnancies are at risk of neurological damage and cerebral palsy, but the risk in monochorionic pregnancies is three times higher than that in dichorionic pregnancies. There are several postulated mechanisms for cerebral damage, namely:

- hypotension due to massive blood loss into the dead twin's placenta
- vascular occlusion due to thrombi that pass from the dead twin's circulation and affect small cerebral vessels
- haemorrhage resulting from coagulation disorders stimulated by thromboplastins from the dead twin's circulation.

Other organs such as the kidney may be affected in a similar manner and renal failure ensues in the neonatal period. The timing between intrauterine death and organ damage occurring is variable. In some instances, cerebral complications in the co-twin may even predate fetal demise.

The death of one twin *in utero* will usually stimulate uterine activity and most pregnancies will deliver within three weeks of the death occurring. As intrauterine death most commonly happens in the late second trimester, many of these pregnancies will deliver prematurely, compounding the problems of the surviving co-twin.

MATERNAL COMPLICATIONS

Maternal coagulation disorders may occur when a dead twin is retained *in utero* for a prolonged period of time. Where delivery is not planned for several weeks, in order to achieve reasonable fetal maturity for the co-twin, weekly coagulation screens should be performed.

MANAGEMENT

Where the intrauterine death of one twin occurs beyond 34 weeks of gestation, delivery of the surviving twin should be planned. Prior to this, most would advocate administration of antenatal steroids and, if fetal monitoring were satisfactory, conservative management of the pregnancy until around 34 weeks of gestation. While there is no clear evidence that mode of delivery affects the outcome of the surviving twin, many of these pregnancies are delivered by caesarean section.

Fetal growth and growth discordancy

Clinical estimation of fetal size in a twin pregnancy is inaccurate and it is impossible by clinical examination alone to detect a growth discrepancy between twins. In most centres ultrasound examination is now used to evaluate fetal size, although repeated studies have confirmed that ultrasound may underestimate or overestimate fetal weight by as much as 10%, a similar margin of error as in singleton pregnancies.

Discordant fetal growth is defined as an inter-twin weight difference of greater than 20% and may be found in 10–30% of all twin pregnancies. While perinatal mortality is reported to be higher in discordant twins, it should not be the only risk factor evaluated. Dizygotic twins, having completely distinct genetic material, will have different growth potentials and may well demonstrate discordant growth patterns but be healthy. Alternatively, both twins may be growth-restricted and show no growth discordancy. For this reason, serial growth scans to evaluate growth velocity and assess amniotic fluid and fetal movements are more widely used to detect those fetuses which, irrespective of size, are compromised *in utero*. As in a singleton pregnancy, when the growth velocity is falling significantly or the estimated fetal weight is less than the fifth centile for gestational age and the liquor volume is reduced, close fetal monitoring should be instigated. This may include umbilical artery Doppler measurements and cardiotocography.

Complications of monochorionic twin pregnancies

TWIN-TO-TWIN TRANSFUSION SYNDROME

On close examination, nearly all monochorionic placentas demonstrate vascular connections. The majority of these are superficial arterioarterial or venovenous vessels that run within the chorionic plate and have little effect on the haemodynamic status of either twin. These twins are likely to be appropriately grown and reach a viable gestation. A small percentage of monochorionic twin placentas, however, possess direct arteriovenous connections that exist deep within the body of the placental mass. Frequently, these connections do not fit a clear line of demarcation, such that the arterial area perfused by one twin may well be larger than the venous area that it drains. In such circumstances the co-twin will

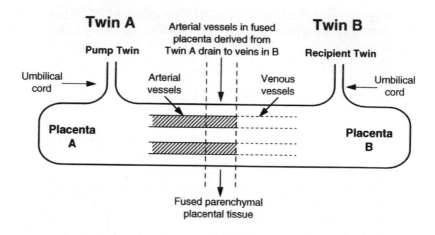

Figure 9.5 Proposed mechanism for the development of twin-to-twin transfusion syndrome

receive an extra load of venous blood (Figure 9.5). In the absence of a large number of connecting superficial vessels to return the extra venous blood, unidirectional transfusion occurs, with one twin as a perfusing donor and the other as a recipient. The donor twin soon becomes hypovolaemic and blood flow to vital organs such as the heart and brain is preserved at the expense of more peripheral structures. Renal perfusion is therefore reduced and urine production diminished. Oligohydramnios ensues in the amniotic sac of the donor twin. The recipient twin, in contrast, has an excess vascular volume. To compensate for this, urine production increases and polyhydramnios develops. This sequence of events is known as twin-to-twin transfusion syndrome or oligopolyhydramnios sequence.

TTTS usually occurs between 18 and 24 weeks of gestation and without intervention is almost universally fatal. Over a five-year period at the Queen Mother's Hospital, Glasgow, 46% of perinatal deaths in monochorionic twins were a direct consequence of TTTS. The high mortality rate is due both to the direct effects of vascular volume changes in both twins and the extreme preterm labour and delivery that occurs as a consequence of massive polyhydramnios. Several treatment options are currently under investigation; namely, serial amniocentesis with or without septostomy (Figure 9.6), laser ablation of the placental vascular connections and indomethacin therapy. Indomethacin does not appear to reduce the polyhydramnios of TTTS sufficiently to prevent preterm labour and it compounds the oliguria of the donor twin, such that complete

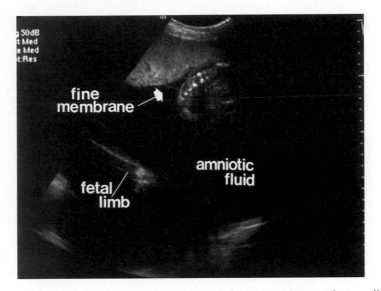

Figure 9.6 Ultrasound of twin-to-twin transfusion syndrome; the small twin is stuck in a corner of the uterus with only a tiny potion of membrane identified due to the oligohydramnios; the recipient twin is surrounded by large pools of amniotic fluid

neonatal anuria may occur. Laser ablation of placental vessels and serial amniocentesis are both widely used. A European randomised study comparing both modalities is currently in progress. Individual centres have reported survival rates of 40–60% with both techniques but these figures are based on small numbers. Cerebral white-matter lesions are present in around 30% of survivors. These lesions are associated with impaired intellectual development in some children.

TWIN REVERSE ARTERIAL PERFUSION SEQUENCE/ACARDIAC TWIN

On rare occasions, one normal twin will develop with an abnormal twin that has no independent cardiac activity (acardiac twin). In many instances these pregnancies miscarry or the acardiac fetus is reabsorbed. If, however, the cord insertions of both twins are closely apposed and there are large direct arterioarterial and venovenous connections between the two pregnancies, the normal twin will perfuse both circulations successfully. The normal (pump) twin is at significant risk of cardiac failure and up to 50% will die *in utero*. Acardiac twins appear grossly abnormal (Figure 9.7 a,b) and frequently only a torso and remnants of the

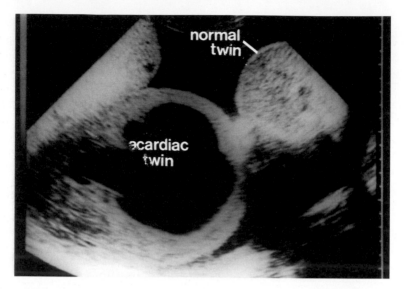

Figure 9.7a Twin reverse arterial perfusion sequence: transabdominal ultrasound image of a large acardiac twin in transverse section at 28 weeks of gestation; an abdominal cross-section of the normal twin is also seen in this image illustrating the massive size discrepancy

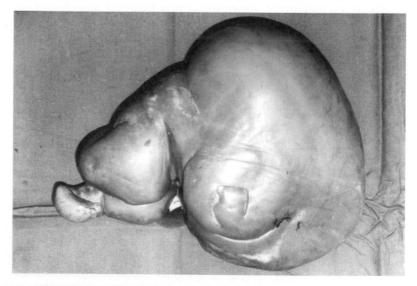

Figure 9.7b Twin reverse arterial perfusion sequence: the acardiac twin shown in Figure 9.7a after delivery three weeks later

lower limbs remain. The exact mechanism for this unusual scenario is unclear. It is possible that the acardiac twin is abnormal from the time of conception and only 'grows' as a result of the cardiac output it receives from the pump twin. Alternatively, the twin pregnancy may begin normally but with time one twin dominates the circulation of the other and arterial blood is pumped via the arterial connections through the umbilical arteries of the second twin (reversed perfusion). Since the retrograde blood flowing through the recipient twin is hypoxic and contains large amounts of waste products, it may well induce ischaemic damage with necrosis in some areas.

Treatment for this problem is limited. Where there is evidence of cardiac failure in the pump twin, selective termination of the acardiac twin has been attempted using thrombogenic coils or cord ligation. A conservative approach is generally advocated if the acardiac twin is small and/or there is no evidence of failure in the normal twin. As the circulation of the normal twin is vulnerable, even minor insults such as uterine contractions may not be tolerated. Once a reasonable gestation is reached, 'elective' delivery by caesarean section is often indicated.

CONJOINT TWINS

Conjoint twins are a rare phenomenon, occurring in only one in 200 000 live births. The complication arises when the zygote divides after 12 days of gestation (Figure 9.8). Conjoint twins are described according to their main site of fusion, the most common being thoracopagus (40%), followed by omphalopagus (33%) and pyopagus (20%), with pelvic

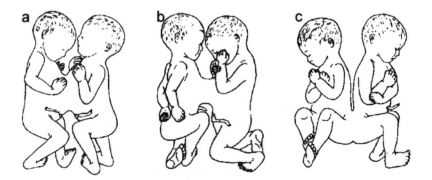

Figure 9.8 Examples of conjoint twinning (a) both chest and thorax fused (b) chest fusion – thoracopagus (c) pelvic fusion – ischiopagus

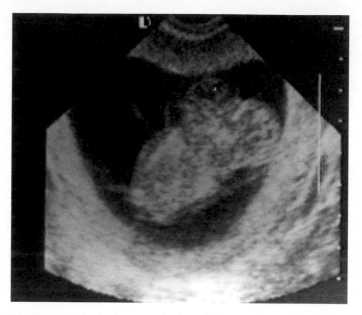

Figure 9.9 Transvaginal ultrasound of conjoint twins at ten weeks of gestation; the twins were joined at the chest and abdomen but two independent heartbeats were eventually identified

(ischiopagus) and cranial (craniopagus) fusion occurring infrequently. Immediate survival and successful separation depend largely on the degree of union and the organs involved. Where the heart or cardiac connections are shared, division is virtually impossible. Attempts have been made to separate affected twins by sacrificing one twin in order to maintain cardiac anatomy and functions in the other but to date there are few long-term survivors. Major blood loss complicates most attempts at separation, which is due in part to the vascular nature of the organs being divided and the extensive vascular connections that exist between both twins.

Conjoint twins should be diagnosed prenatally by ultrasound and the area of fusion identified (Figure 9.9). When the diagnosis is made early, parents may opt to terminate the pregnancy. Those who choose to continue with the pregnancy should be delivered by caesarean section in a tertiary unit with appropriate obstetric, neonatal and paediatric staff available.

Long-term outcome of twin pregnancies

The incidence of cerebral palsy is consistently three to five times higher among twin pregnancies. Death of a co-twin *in utero* is significantly associated with neurodevelopmental problems. As most of the studies to date have not recorded zygosity or chorionicity, it is not clear if cerebral palsy is strongly correlated with either of these groups. Neonatal and non-febrile seizures are reported to be more frequent among monozygotic twins. Since many twins deliver prematurely, the excess of cerebral palsy in twins has been attributed by some to preterm delivery. However, several studies confirm that preterm twin pregnancies still demonstrate an increased incidence of learning difficulties even when matched with singleton pregnancies delivered at a similar gestation.

Summary

Twin pregnancies continue to present a management challenge to clinicians. It is hoped that as the problems that complicate these pregnancies are more thoroughly understood, antenatal care may be targeted and preventive strategies developed to reduce long-term perinatal morbidity and mortality.

References

Barlow DH, Mahmud G. (1995) Assisted conception and multiple pregnancy. In: Ward RH, Whittle M, editors. *Multiple Pregnancy*. London: RCOG Press. p. 30–8.

Finberg HJ. (1992) The 'twin-peak' sign: reliable evidence of dichorionic twinning. *J Ultrasound Med* **11**:571–7.

Neilson JP, Verkuyl DAA, Crowther CA, Bannerman C. (1988). Preterm labour in twin pregnancies: prediction by cervical assessment. *Obstet Gynaecol* **72**:719–23.

Newman RB, Godsey RK, Ellings JM, Campbell BA, Eller DP, Miller MC. (1991) Quantification of cervical change: relationship to preterm delivery in the multifetal gestation. *Am J Obstet Gynecol* **165**:264–71.

Quintero RA, Johnson MP, Reich H, Goncalves L, Johnson MP, Carreno C, *et al.* (1996) *In utero* percutaneous umbilical cord ligation in the management of complicated monochorionic multiple gestations. *J Ultrasound Obstet Gynaecol* **8**:16–22.

Sebire NJ, Snijders RJM, Hughes K, Sepulveda W, Nicolaides KH. (1996) Screening for trisomy 21 in twin pregnancies by maternal age and fetal nuchal translucency at 10–14 weeks of gestation. *Br J Obstet Gynaecol* **103**:999–1003.

Sepulveda W, Seibre NJ, Hughes K, Odibo A, Nicolaides KH. (1996) The lambda sign at 10–14 weeks gestation as a predictor of chorionicity in twin pregnancies. *Ultrasound Obstet Gynaecol* **7**:421–3.

Tabor A, Philip J, Madsen M, Bang J, Obel EB, Norgaard-Pedersen B. (1986) Randomised controlled trial of genetic amniocentesis in 4606 low-risk women. *Lancet* **i**:1287–93.

Index

A/B ratio 114
abdomen, anomaly scan 28, 30, 35
abdominal wall defects 48, 49–51
abortion *see* miscarriage; termination of
	pregnancy
Abortion Act, 1967 101
acardiac twin 133–5
achondrogenesis 53
achondroplasia 53
adenosine, fetal therapy 58
adrenal hyperplasia,
		congenital (CAH) 57
Afro-Caribbeans,
		Down syndrome screening 4
akinesia syndrome, fetal 92
alpha-fetoprotein (α-FP)
	in abdominal wall defects 48
	Down syndrome screening 2–4
	in other chromosomal
		abnormalities 10
	screening for neural tube defects 42
amniocentesis 13, 15–17
	audit 23–5
	cytogenetic analysis 16
	early (before 14 weeks) 17
	in hydrops fetalis 92
	in multiple pregnancy 21–2, 129
	in Rhesus disease 60–1
	risks 16
	therapeutic 72–3
	timing 17
	versus chorionic villus sampling 20
amniodrainage 72–3
	in twin-to-twin transfusion
		syndrome 73–4, 79, 133
amnioinfusion 69, 72
amniotic bands, fetoscopic lysis 81

amniotic fluid
	bilirubin levels
		(Delta OD450) 60–1, 63
	leakage, after amniocentesis 17
	volume, in IUGR 113
anaemia, fetal
	cordocentesis 22
	hydrops fetalis 94
	in parvovirus B19 infection 96
	in Rhesus disease 61–2, 64
analgesia
	invasive fetal procedures 82
	termination of pregnancy 104
anencephaly 42, 43
aneuploidies *see*
		chromosomal abnormalities
anomaly scan, routine 27–39
	aims 36
	first trimester 34–6
	'missed' anomalies 38
	problems 36–9
	RCOG recommendations 38
	second trimester 28–34
	in twin pregnancy 128
anti-arrhythmic therapy, fetal 58
anti-D immuno-
		globulin 16, 20, 103, 104
anti-SSA/La autoantibodies 59
anti-SSA/Ro autoantibodies 59
anticoagulant therapy 27
anticonvulsant therapy 27
anxiety, routine anomaly scanning 39
aortic blood flow, in IUGR fetus 116
aortic stenosis 48
aplastic crisis, parvovirus B19
		infection 95, 98
Arnold–Chiari malformation 43, 78

arrhythmias, fetal 57–9, 91
arthrogryposis multiplex 92
ascites, fetal 88, 93
  urinary 69
aspirin, in IUGR prevention 120
assisted conception 123
atrial ectopic beats, fetal 59
atrioventricular septal defects 47, 48
audit
  fetoscopic procedures 81
  invasive prenatal diagnostic
    procedures 23–5
awareness, fetal 81–2

Ballantyne (maternal mirror)
    syndrome 77, 93
'banana' sign 43
β-human chorionic
    gonadotrophin (βhCG)
  Down syndrome
    screening 3, 4–5, 8, 9
  in other chromosomal
    abnormalities 10
bilirubin, amniotic fluid
    (Delta OD450) 60–1, 63
biochemical screening
  Down syndrome *see* Down
    syndrome, biochemical screening
  other chromosomal
    abnormalities 10
bladder drainage, fetal 68–9
blood volume, fetal-placental 64, 65
body stalk anomaly 51
bowel, echogenic 37
bradycardia, fetal
  after cordocentesis 23
  after intravascular transfusion 65
  hydrops fetalis 91
  medical therapy 59
bromocriptine 104
bronchopulmonary
    sequestration 76–7

cardiotocography (CTG),
    in IUGR 111–13
cardiovascular disease
  in adult life, after IUGR 121

fetal 91
  in growth-restricted infant 118
  see also arrhythmias, fetal; congenital
    heart disease
central nervous system,
    congenital abnormalities 42–5
cerebral blood flow,
    in IUGR fetus 115–16
cerebral haemorrhage,
    growth-restricted neonate 118
cerebral palsy
  after IUGR 118
  in twins 130, 136–7
cervical length, predicting
    preterm labour 126–7
chest, fetal
  abnormalities causing hydrops 91
  anomaly scan 28, 30
chorionic villus sampling
    (CVS) 9, 13, 17–21
  audit 23–5
  contraindications 20
  cytogenetic analysis 21
  in hydrops fetalis 92
  in multiple pregnancy 21–2
  risks 21
  techniques 18–20
  timing 18
  in twin pregnancy 129
  versus amniocentesis 20
chorionicity of twin pregnancy 123–6
  prenatal determination 124–5
  value of determining 125–6
  see also monochorionic twin
    pregnancy
choroid plexus
  cysts 36–7
  first trimester appearance 34, 35
chromosomal abnormalities
  congenital heart disease 47, 48
  in gastrointestinal
    anomalies 48, 50, 51
  hydrops fetalis 90
  IUGR 109
  prenatal diagnosis 16
  screening 1–11
  soft markers 5, 6, 36–7

in twin pregnancy 128–9
see also Down syndrome
chronic granulomatous disease 82
chylothorax, fetal 70, 91
CLASP trial 120
coagulation disorders, maternal 130
congenital adrenal hyperplasia
    (CAH) 57
congenital cystic adenomatoid
    malformation
    (CCAM) 76–7, 91
congenital diaphragmatic hernia
    (CDH) 51, 74–6
congenital heart disease (CHD)
  antenatal detection 45–8
  associated anomalies 47, 48
  in Down syndrome 5
  hydrops fetalis 91
  parental 27
  risk factors 46
congenital infections *see* infections, fetal
congenital malformations *see* fetal
    structural abnormalities
conjoint twins 135–6
consent, for prenatal diagnosis 14
cordocentesis 13, 22–3
  complications 23
  in hydrops fetalis 92
  in parvovirus B19 infection 97
  techniques 22–3
Cornelia de Lange syndrome 92
coronary blood flow, IUGR fetus 117
counselling
  Down syndrome screening 1, 14
  in fetal structural anomalies 53–4
  in hydrops fetalis 92
  prenatal diagnosis 14
  in Rhesus disease 62
  termination of pregnancy for fetal
    abnormality 101
craniopagus 136
CVS *see* chorionic villus sampling
cyclo-oxygenase
    (COX)-2-antagonists 73
cystic adenomatoid malformation,
    congenital (CCAM) 76–7, 91
cystoscopy, fetal, posterior urethral

valve ablation 69
cytogenetic analysis 16, 21
cytotrophoblast 110

dexamethasone,
  maternal therapy 57, 59
diabetes mellitus
  congenital abnormalities 27
  Down syndrome screening 4
diamorphine 104
diaphragmatic hernia,
  congenital (CDH) 51, 74–6
diastolic 'notch' 119, 120
dichorionic twin pregnancy 123, 124–5
digoxin, fetal therapy 58, 94
dilatation and evacuation (D&E) 102
discordant fetal growth, in twin
    pregnancy 131
Donald, Ian 55
Doppler ultrasound 113–14
  in intrauterine transfusion 62, Plate 3
  in IUGR 113–15
  prediction of IUGR 118–20
  in Rhesus disease 61–2, Plate 3
  umbilical artery
    waveforms 113, 114–15
'double bubble' sign 50, 51
double test, Down syndrome
    screening 4
Down syndrome (trisomy 21) 1–10
  biochemical screening 2–5, 13–14
    first trimester 4–5
    and nuchal translucency 8, 9
    second trimester 2–5
    in twin pregnancy 4, 129
  first- versus second-trimester
    screening 9–10
  'high-risk' screening result 1, 14
  hydrops fetalis 90
  maternal age-based
    screening 2, 3, 5, 9, 14
  prenatal diagnosis 13–14
  structural
    abnormalities 5–6, 47, 48, 51
  in twin pregnancy 129
  ultrasound screening 5–8, 14
    first trimester 6–8

second trimester 5–6
  soft markers 5, 6, 37
  in twin pregnancy 129
drugs, fetal therapy 56–7
duodenal atresia 50, 51
dysrrhythmias, fetal 57–9, 91

Ebstein's anomaly 48
echocardiography, fetal
  in arrhythmias 57, 58, 59
  in cardiac anomalies 47
  in hydrops fetalis 91
echogenic bowel 37
encephalocele 42, 44, Plate 1
endoscopes, for fetoscopy 78–9
erythema infectiosum 95
erythropoietin 117
ethics, fetal therapy 83–4
exomphalos 48, 49–50

face, anomaly scan 28, 29, 31
femur length, short 37
fetal abnormality
  late diagnosis 104
  structural see fetal structural
    abnormalities
  termination of pregnancy see
    termination of pregnancy, for
    fetal abnormality
  in twin pregnancy 128–9
fetal akinesia syndrome 92
fetal blood sampling
  in hydrops fetalis 92
  for prenatal diagnosis 13, 22–3
fetal heart rate variability,
    in IUGR 111–13
fetal loss
  amniocentesis 16, 17
  chorionic villus sampling 21
  cordocentesis 23
  parvovirus B19 infection 95
  selective termination 106, 128
  see also miscarriage
fetal structural abnormalities 41–54
  aetiology 41
  cardiovascular system 45–8
  central nervous system 42–5

chorionic villus sampling
  and 17–18, 21
  in chromosomal abnormalities 10
  in Down syndrome 5–6, 47, 48, 51
  frequency 41
  gastrointestinal system 49–51
  in utero surgery see fetal surgery
  IUGR 109
  maternal risk factors 27
  missed 38
  prevention 55–6
  renal tract abnormalities 51–2
  routine anomaly scan 27–39
  skeletal system 53
  in twin pregnancy 128–9
fetal surgery 36, 73–81
  minimally invasive 78–81
  'open' 73–8
  potential indications 74
fetal therapy 55–84
  to alter amount of amniotic
    fluid 72–4
  ethics 83–4
  fetal pain and awareness 81–2
  future prospects 82–3
  historical aspects 55
  indirect (transplacental) 56–9
  invasive 59–67
  preventive therapy 55–6
  shunting procedures 67–72
  surgery see fetal surgery
feticide
  late, for fetal abnormality 104–5
  for multifetal pregnancy
    reduction 105–6
  selective
    acardiac twin 135
    for fetal
      abnormality 104–8, 128
    monochorionic
      twins 80–1, 107–8, 128
fetomaternal alloimmune
    thrombocytopenia (FMAIT) 66–7
fetomaternal haemorrhage 94
fetoscopy 78–81
  complications of operative 81
  cord occlusion in monochorionic

twins 80–1, 107–8, 128
laser ablation of placental
   vessels 79–80, 133
laser ablation of posterior urethral
   valves 69
lysis of amniotic bands 81
fibronectin, fetal (FFN) 126
fifth disease 95
first trimester
   abortion for fetal abnormality 101–2
   anomaly scan 34–6
   chorionicity determination 124–5
   Down syndrome
      screening 4–5, 6–8, 9–10
   prenatal diagnosis 9, 17
flecainide, fetal therapy 58
flow velocity waveform (FVW) 114
fluorescence *in situ* hybridisation (FISH)
   16
folic acid supplements 45, 56
foot, anomaly scan 33
fractures, *in utero* 53

gastrointestinal system, congenital
   anomalies 49–51
gastroschisis 48, 49–50, Plate 2
gemeprost 102, 103
gene therapy 83
genetic diseases
   gene therapy 83
   hydrops fetalis 92
genital tract infection, post-abortion 102
glucose-6-phosphate dehydrogenase
   deficiency 94
granulomatous disease, chronic 82
growth, fetal
   discordant, in twin pregnancy 131
   in twin pregnancy 131
   see also intrauterine growth restriction

haematocrit
   donor blood 65
   fetal 64, 65
   growth-restricted neonate 118
haemoglobinopathies, fetal stem cell
   transplantation 82
haemorrhage

complicating abortion 102
   fetomaternal 94
'halo' sign 88
hand, anomaly scan 29
head, anomaly scan 28, 31
heart
   anomaly scan 30
   echogenic foci 37
heart block, complete 59
heart disease, congenital *see* congenital
   heart disease
heat loss, growth-restricted
   neonate 118
human chorionic gonadotrophin (hCG)
   in chromosomal abnormalities 3–4, 10
   free β-subunit *see* β-human chorionic
      gonadotrophin
human parvovirus B19 infection *see*
   parvovirus B19 infection
humerus, short 6
hydrocephalus 45, 118
hydronephrosis 52
hydrops fetalis Plate 2
   in arrhythmias 58, 59, 91
   in congenital cystic adenomatoid
      malformation (CCAM) 76, 91
   non-immune (NIH) 87–98, Plate 6
      aetiology 90–8
      fetal anaemia 94
      genetic causes 92
      infectious 94
      investigation and
         management 87, 89, 92–4
      non-infectious 92–4
      parvovirus B19 infection 94–8
      prenatal diagnosis 87, 88
   in parvovirus
      B19 infection 96, 97, Plate 7
   pleural effusions 71, 88, 93
   in Rhesus disease 60
   in sacrococcygeal teratoma 77
hypertension, in adult life,
   after IUGR 121
hypertonic saline 102
hypoglycaemia, growth-restricted
   neonate 118
hypoplastic left-heart syndrome

(HLHS) 47–8
hypoxia, chronic fetal 116, 117
    see also intrauterine growth restriction

imaging, fetal 55
immunodeficiency, fetal stem cell
        transplantation 82
immunoglobulin, intravenous 67
inborn errors of metabolism,
        maternal 56
indomethacin 72, 132–3
infections, fetal
    investigations 92
    IUGR 109
    management 94
    see also parvovirus B19 infection
inhibin A 3, 4
insulin-like growth factor-I (IGF-I) 121
intraperitoneal transfusion 60, 62
intrauterine death (IUD)
        of one twin 129–31
    complications in
            surviving twin 130, 136–7
    management 130–1
    maternal complications 130
intrauterine growth restriction
        (IUGR) 109–21
    amniotic fluid volume 113
    antenatal features 111–15
    causes 109
    in congenital heart disease 48
    fetal blood flow distribution 115–17
    fetal metabolism 117
    long-term sequelae 121
    neonatal effects 117–18
    potential therapies 120–1
    prediction from uterine artery
            Doppler 118–20
    in twin pregnancy 131
    unexplained 109
intrauterine transfusion
    intraperitoneal 60, 62
    intravascular 62–5, 66
    in parvovirus B19 infection 97
    in Rhesus disease 60, 62–5

intravascular transfusion,
        in Rhesus disease 62–5, 66
intravenous immunoglobulin 67
ischiopagus 136
IUGR *see* intrauterine growth restriction

Jeune syndrome 91

karyotyping
    chorionic villus sampling for 9, 21
    in congenital heart disease 47
    cordocentesis for 22
    in fetal pleural effusion 71
    in gastrointestinal
            anomalies 48, 50, 51
kidney, anomaly scan 33
kidney disease
    cystic 51, 52
    multicystic 51, 52
    polycystic 45, 51, 52

lactation, suppression of 104
lambda sign 124, 125
laser ablation, fetoscopic
    placental vessels 79–80, 133
    posterior urethral valves 69
'lemon' sign 43, 44
Liggins GC 55
Liley AW 55, 60
Liley curve 60–1, 63
limb-reduction defects, after chorionic
        villus sampling 17,18
limbs, anomaly scan 28, 29, 33
liver
    cells, *in utero* transplantation 82
    herniation into chest 74–6
local anaesthesia, chorionic villus
        sampling (CVS) 19
lung lesions, fetal 76–7

magnetic resonance imaging (MRI), fetal
    congenital diaphragmatic hernia 76
    sacrococcygeal teratoma 77, 78
maternal age
    Down syndrome
            screening 2, 3, 5, 9, 14
    nuchal translucency and 7, 9

maternal 'mirror' syndrome 77, 93
maternal weight, in Down syndrome
  screening 4
Meckel–Gruber syndrome 45
medical fetal therapy 56–7
metabolic disorders, maternal 56
metabolism, IUGR fetus 117
middle cerebral artery
  flow velocity in IUGR fetus 115–16
  peak systolic velocity
    (PSV) 61–2, 64, Plate 3
mifepristone 102–3
minimally invasive fetal surgery 78–81
'mirror' syndrome, maternal 77, 93
miscarriage
  first-trimester screening and 9
  selective termination 106, 128
  see also fetal loss
misoprostol 102, 103–4
monochorionic twin
    pregnancy 123, 124
  complications 131–6
  cord occlusion for selective
    feticide 80–1, 107–8, 128
  fetal abnormality 128
  intrauterine death of one twin 130
  invasive prenatal testing 129
  nuchal translucency 129
  prenatal determination 124–5
  twin-to-twin transfusion
    syndrome 73, 79, 131–3
  value of prenatal detection 125–6
mosaicism 10, 21
mucopolysaccharidoses 92
multicystic kidney disease 51, 52
multifetal pregnancy reduction 105–8
multiple pregnancy
  Down syndrome screening 4, 129
  fetal reduction 105–6
  invasive diagnostic
    techniques 21–2, 129
  see also twin pregnancy
multiples of the median (MOM) 2–3
myelomeningocele 43, Plate 1
  in utero surgery 77–8
myotonic dystrophy 92

necrotising enterocolitis 116
neonates, growth-restricted 117–18
Neu Laxova syndrome 92
neural tube defects 42–5
  associated anomalies 44–5
  in utero surgery 77–8
  prevention 45, 55–6
  risk factors 42
  screening 42
neurological sequelae
  intrauterine death of
    co-twin 130, 136–7
  IUGR 118
  twin-to-twin transfusion
    syndrome 73, 80, 133
  see also cerebral palsy
non-disjunction 2
Noonan syndrome 92
'notch', diastolic 119, 120
nuchal fold thickness, Down
    syndrome 5–6
nuchal translucency (NT) 5–8
  in Down syndrome screening 8, 9
  measurement 6–7
  miscarriage and 9
  in monochorionic twin
    pregnancy 129
  in multifetal pregnancy
    reduction 106
  in other chromosomal
    abnormalities 10
nutrient supplementation,
    in IUGR 120–1

oestriol, unconjugated (uE$_3$) 3–4
oligohydramnios 51–2
  amnioinfusion 72
  in twin-to-twin transfusion
    syndrome 132, 133
  in urinary tract obstruction 69
oligopolyhydramnios sequence see
    twin-to-twin transfusion
    syndrome
omphalopagus 135
orthopaedic problems, after
    amniocentesis 16, 17
osteogenesis imperfecta 53

oxygen administration, in IUGR 120–1

pain, fetal 81–2
parvovirus B19 infection 94–8, Plate 6
  clinical features 95
  effect on pregnancy 95–6
  management 97
  population screening 97–8
pelviureteric obstruction 52
Pena–Shokeir syndrome 92
perinatal medicine 55
periventricular leucomalacia 118
persistent fetal circulation 118
pharmacokinetics, fetal 56–7
phenylketonuria (PKU),
  maternal 27, 56
placenta
  blood vessels 111, Plate 8
  drug transfer 56–7
  normal development 110–11
placental vessels, fetoscopic laser
  ablation 79–80, 133
platelet antigens, maternal
  alloimmunisation 67
platelet transfusion, fetal 67
pleural effusions, fetal 70–2
  drainage 71–2, 93
  hydrops fetalis 71, 88, 91, 93
pleuroamniotic
  shunting 71–2, 93, Plate 4
PLUG technique, congenital
  diaphragmatic hernia 76
polycystic kidney disease 45, 51, 52
polycythaemia, growth-restricted
  neonate 118
polyhydramnios
  amniodrainage 73
  in twin-to-twin transfusion
    syndrome 132, 133
posterior urethral valves
  (PUV) 52, 67–9
  fetal cystoscopic ablation 69
  vesicoamniotic shunting 67–8, 69–70
postmortem examination 54, 92
potassium chloride, intracardiac
  injection
  for late termination 104

for multifetal pregnancy
  reduction 105, 106
for selective feticide 107, 128
pregnancy-associated plasma protein A
  (PAPP-A) 4–5, 8, 9
prenatal diagnosis 13–25
  audit 23–5
  first trimester 9
  first-trimester screening and 9–10
  indications 13–14
  in multiple pregnancy 21–2
  non-immune hydrops fetalis 87, 88
  techniques 13
  in twin pregnancy 129
  see also amniocentesis; chorionic villus
    sampling; cordocentesis
prepregnancy advice 55–6
preterm delivery, twin pregnancy 126
preterm labour
  prediction 126–8
  treatment 128
  in twin pregnancy 126
preterm prelabour rupture of the
  membranes (PPROM) 72, 81
prostaglandin synthetase inhibitors 72
prostaglandins
  first-trimester abortion 101
  mid-trimester abortion 102, 103–4
'prune belly' syndrome 67, Plate 4
psychological effects
  late diagnosis of fetal abnormality 104
  routine anomaly scanning 39
pulmonary hypertension,
  in growth-restricted neonate 118
pulmonary hypoplasia 72, 74, 75
pulsatility index (PI) 114
pyopagus 135

quadruple test,
  Down syndrome screening 3

renal agenesis, bilateral 52
renal dysplasia
  cystic 51
  secondary to obstruction 52, 68
renal pyelectasis (renal pelvis
  dilatation) 6, 37

renal tract *see* urinary tract
resistance index (RI) 114
retinoic acid therapy 27
rhesus (Rh) isoimmunisation 60–7
    assessment of fetal
        disease 13, 22, 60–2, 63
    developments in management 60, 61
    intraperitoneal transfusion 60, 62
    intravascular transfusion 62–5, 66
    management algorithm 66
    prevention 16, 20, 103, 104
Royal College of Obstetricians and
    Gynaecologists (RCOG),
    guidelines on anomaly
    scanning 38

S/D ratio 114
sacrococcygeal teratoma 77
scalp oedema, in hydrops fetalis 88
screening
    chromosomal abnormalities 1–11
    Down syndrome *see* Down syndrome
    neural tube defects 42
    parvovirus B19 susceptibility 97–8
    see also anomaly scan, routine
second trimester
    abortion for fetal abnormality 102–4
    chorionicity determination 125
    Down syndrome
        screening 2–4, 5–6, 9–10
    prenatal diagnosis 17
    routine anomaly scan 28–34
seizures, neonatal, in twins 137
sex aneuploidies 10
shunting procedures, fetal 67–72
sickle cell disease 82
skeletal dysplasias 53, 91
'slapped cheek' syndrome 95, Plate 7
small for gestational age (SGA) 109
    see also intrauterine growth restriction
smoking,
    Down syndrome screening and 4
soft markers
    Down syndrome 5, 6, 37
    routine anomaly scans 36–7
spina bifida 42, 43–4, Plate 1
    in utero surgery 77–8

parental 27
spine, anomaly scan 28, 32
spiral arteries, trophoblast
    invasion 110, 111, 120
stem cell transplantation,
    in utero 81, 82
structural malformations *see* fetal
    structural abnormalities
substrate supplementation,
    in IUGR 120–1
supraventricular tachycardia (SVT),
    fetal 57–8, 91
syncytiotrophoblast 110
systemic circulation, in IUGR fetus 116

T sign 125
tachycardia, fetal 57–8, 90, 91
talipes, after amniocentesis 16, 17
teratoma, sacrococcygeal 77
termination of pregnancy
    for fetal abnormality 54, 101–8
        after first-trimester screening 9
        after routine anomaly
        scan 36, 38, 39
        first trimester 101–2
        late 104–5
        mid-trimester 102–4
        in multiple pregnancy 106–8
    in hydrops fetalis 93
    legal basis 101
    selective *see* feticide, selective
α-thalassaemia 94
β-thalassaemia 82
thanatophoric dysplasia
    (dwarfism) 53, 91
thermoregulation, growth-restricted
    neonate 118
thoracic dysplasia, asphyxiating 91
thoracoamniotic shunt 71–2, 76, Plate 4
thoracocentesis, fetal 71
thoracopagus 135
thorax, fetal *see* chest, fetal
thrombocytopenia, fetomaternal
    alloimmune (FMAIT) 66–7

tocolysis, in twin pregnancy 128
tracheal occlusion, in congenital
        diaphragmatic hernia 76
transfusion, fetal *see* intrauterine
        transfusion
translocations, unbalanced 10
transvaginal ultrasound,
        anomaly scan 35–6
triple test,
        Down syndrome screening 4
triploidy 10, 90
trisomy 13
    hydrops fetalis 90
    screening 10
    structural abnormalities 47, 48
trisomy 16, 90
trisomy 18
    hydrops fetalis 90
    screening 10
    structural
        abnormalities 37, 44, 47, 48
trisomy 21 *see* Down syndrome
trophoblast invasion 110–11, 120
Turner syndrome (45XO) 10
    hydrops fetalis 90
    structural abnormalities 47, 48
twin pregnancy 123–37
    chorionicity and zygosity 123–6
    dichorionic 123, 124–5
    Down syndrome screening 4, 129
    fetal abnormality 128–9
    fetal growth and growth
        discordancy 131
    intrauterine death of
        one twin 129–31
    long-term outcome 136–7
    monochorionic *see* monochorionic
        twin pregnancy
    predicting preterm labour 126–8
    preterm delivery 126
    selective termination 106–8
    treatment of preterm labour 128
    see also multiple pregnancy
twin reversed arterial perfusion (TRAP)
        sequence 80, 133–5

twin-to-twin transfusion syndrome
        (TTTS) 73–4, 131–3, Plate 5
    laser ablation of placental vessels
        79–80, 133
    serial amniodrainage 73, 80, 133
twins
    acardiac 133–5
    conjoint 135–6
    dizygous (non-identical) 123–4
    intrauterine death of one 129–31
    monozygous (identical) 123–4

ultrasound
    cervical length assessment 127
    in chorionicity determination 124–5
    Down syndrome
        screening 5–8, 9, 14, 129
    -guided amniocentesis 15
    -guided chorionic villus sampling 19
    -guided cordocentesis 22–3
    -guided invasive fetal therapy 59–67
    in hydrops fetalis 87, 88, 92
    in IUGR 111, 112
    in neural tube defects 42
    in Rhesus disease 60
    routine anomaly scan 27–39
    screening for chromosomal
        abnormalities 10
    see also Doppler ultrasound;
        echocardiography, fetal
umbilical artery
        Doppler studies 113, 114–15
umbilical cord occlusion,
        in complicated monochorionic
        twins 80–1, 107–8, 128
umbilical vein
    blood sampling 22–3
    intrauterine transfusion 63–5
urea 102
urethral valves, posterior *see* posterior
        urethral valves
urinary tract
    abnormalities 51–2
    obstruction, fetal 52, 67–9

urine
  output, IUGR fetus 116
  sampling, fetal 68–9
uterine activity monitoring,
      in twin pregnancy 127–8
uterine artery Doppler,
      prediction of IUGR 118–20
uterine perforation,
      complicating abortion 102
uteroplacental development
  in IUGR 111
  normal 109–11
uteroplacental insufficiency 109, 111

vacuum aspiration,
      termination of pregnancy 101–2
ventricular septal defects 48
vesicoamniotic
      shunting 52, 67–70, Plate 4
  procedure 69–70
  results 69
  selection for 68–9
vesicocentesis 68

warfarin therapy 27
weight, maternal,
      in Down syndrome screening 4
Wilson's disease, maternal 56

zygosity of twin pregnancy 123–4

PUBLISHED TITLES IN THE MRCOG & BEYOND SERIES

All titles in this series are available from the RCOG Bookshop

Tel: +44 (0) 20 7772 6275;
fax: +44 (0) 20 7724 5991;
email: bookshop@rcog.org.uk
Buy online at **www.rcog.org.uk**

Intrapartum Care for the MRCOG and Beyond

Thomas F Baskett and Sabatnam Arulkumaran

Pregnancy and childbirth carry risks for the mother and to her baby. Worldwide, some 600 000 maternal deaths are recorded each year, of which 99% occur in developing countries, while many developed countries record low maternal mortality rates of about six per 100 000 and perinatal mortality rates of 6–8 per 1000.

There are still avoidable factors in many maternal and perinatal deaths. There are around 20–30 near-miss cases per maternal death. Similarly, the perinatal risk is greatest during labour and delivery and standards of perinatal care can be assessed by reviews of perinatal mortality and morbidity, including asphyxia, trauma and infection.

This book provides a balanced but pragmatic guide to clinical intrapartum care. It is an invaluable aid, not only for candidates preparing to sit the MRCOG examination but also for those in clinical practice, midwives and, indeed, any health professional who comes into contact with mothers.

Contents: Preface; Abbreviations; Introduction; First stage of labour; second stage of labour; Fetal surveillance in labour; Third stage of labour; Induction of labour; Preterm labour and prelabour rupture of membranes; Assisted vaginal delivery; Breech vaginal delivery; Twin and triplet delivery; Caesarean section; Vaginal birth after caesarean section; Uterine rupture and emergency hysterectomy; Shoulder dystocia; Cord prolapse; Antepartum haemorrhage; Postpartum haemorrhage; Amniotic fluid embolism; Severe pre-eclampsia and eclampsia; Neonatal resuscitation by John McIntyre; Perinatal loss by Carolyn Basak; Further reading; Index.

| 1-900364-73-5 | 224 pages | Published 2002 |

Menopause for the MRCOG and Beyond

Margaret Rees

The management of the menopause and hormone replacement therapy has become an increasingly important subject for the MRCOG examinations in recent years. This review provides the MRCOG trainee with an excellent insight and with more than enough current facts and figures, but it will also be extremely useful for anyone else wishing to be up-to-date in this increasingly important area.

Contents: Preface; Introduction, definitions and physiology; Consequences of ovarian failure; Investigations; Benefits of HRT; Risks of HRT; HRT: preparations, prescribing, treatment duration and management of adverse effects; Specific pre-existing medical conditions and HRT; Monitoring HRT; Non-hormone replacement therapy and osteoporosis; Complementary and alternative therapies; Index.

| 1-900364-45-X | 98 pages | Published 2002 |

Paediatric and Adolescent Gynaecology for the MRCOG and Beyond

Anne Garden and Joanne Topping

A broad knowledge of caring for children and adolescents with gynaecological disorders is essential for everyone in clinical practice. All clinicians, at some point in their careers, will be required to deal with young people who present with symptoms that could possibly be due to gynaecological pathology. This book covers the whole range of developments in the field of paediatric and adolescent gynaecology, ranging from conditions specific to childhood to contraception, female genital mutilation and gynaecological malignancies. The subject is dealt with in a sensitive and understanding manner and is clearly written by authors with a worldwide reputation in the field. It is an invaluable aid, not only for candidates preparing to sit the MRCOG examination but also for those in clinical practice, midwives and, indeed, any health professional who comes into contact with young people.

Contents: Preface; Pubertal growth and development; Indeterminate genitalia; Gynaecological problems in childhood; Endocrine disorders; Child sexual abuse; Amenorrhoea; Menstrual problems in teenagers; Contraception; Female genital mutilation; Gynaecological tumours; Index.

1-900364-42-5	96 pages	Published 2001

Antenatal Disorders for the MRCOG and Beyond

Andrew Thompson and Ian Greer

Patterns and provision of antenatal care have changed enormously in recent years in response to the opinions of consumers, providers, professional associations and government reports. During pregnancy, most women remain well and require little formal medical input. For them, pregnancy is a physiological process. However, some women develop complications with significant morbidity or mortality for their baby and, occasionally, for themselves. Providers of antenatal care must be able to distinguish between these two groups of women and arrange with them an appropriate and personalised plan of care.

Contents: Preface; Antenatal care and risk assessment; Assessment of fetal growth and well-being; Antepartum haemorrhage; Multiple pregnancy; Preterm labour; Hypertensive disorders of pregnancy; Common medical disorders in pregnancy; Rhesus disease; Recommended reading; Index.

1-900364-36-0	208 pages	Published 2000

Management of Infertility for the MRCOG and Beyond

Allan Templeton, P Ashok, S Bhattacharya, R Gazvani, M Hamilton, S MacMillan & A Shetty

Every MRCOG candidate must have a broad knowledge of infertility management. This volume has been written jointly by members of one of the most prestigious infertility clinics in the UK (Aberdeen Maternity Hospital) and provides information on all aspects of infertility, both male and female.

Contents: Preface; The management of infertility; The initial assessment of the infertile couple; Male factor infertility; Disorders of ovulation; Tubal-factor infertility; Infertility and endometriosis; Unexplained infertility; Assisted conception techniques; Glossary; Recommended reading; Index.

1-900364-29-8	131 pages	Published 2000

Gynaecological and Obstetric Pathology for the MRCOG

Harold Fox and Hilary Buckley

This succinct and copiously illustrated volume covers pathological conditions of the vulva, vagina, uterus, fallopian tube and ovary, in addition to abnormalities related to pregnancy, and cervical cytology. Gynaecological and Obstetric Pathology is an invaluable revision text for candidates preparing for the Part 1 and Part 2 MRCOG Examination, and is in addition a readily accessible, concise and up-to-date reference text for practising clinicians.

Contents: Preface; The vulva; The vagina; The cervix; The endometrium; The myometrium; The fallopian tube; The ovary; Abnormalities related to pregnancy; Cervical cytology, *by Dulcie V Coleman*; Suggested references for further reading; Index.

0-902331-84-1	184 pages	Published 1998

Menstrual Problems for the MRCOG

Mary Anne Lumsden, Jane Norman and Hilary Critchley

This text covers normal endometrial function, evaluation of the uterine cavity, medical and surgical treatment of menstrual problems, dysmenorrhoea, adolescent bleeding problems, perimenopausal and iatrogenic bleeding.

Contents: Preface; Introduction; Normal endometrial function; Evaluation of the uterine cavity; Medical management of menstrual problems; Surgical treatment of menstrual problems; Dysmenorrhoea; Adolescent bleeding problems; Iatrogenic bleeding; Index.

0-902331-83-3	111 pages	Published 1997

Neonatology for the MRCOG

Peter Dear and Simon Newell

Written with the trainee obstetrician in mind and concentrates on those aspects of the subject that are relevant to obstetric decision making.

Contents: Preface; Introduction; The effects of birth on the fetus; Care of the normal infant; The preterm infant; Intrauterine growth retardation; Nutrition and infant feeding; Jaundice; Common congenital abnormalities; Infection of the fetus and newborn; Blood disorders; Hydrops fetalis; Inborn errors of metabolism; Neonatal effects of maternal disease; Suggested references for further reading; Index.

0-902331-82-5	136 pages	Published 1996

The MRCOG: A Guide to the Examination

IR Johnson, IT Cameron, EJ Owen, P Bowen-Simpkins and JM Rymer

An essential up-to-date guide to the Examination and gives full details of recent changes in its structure and regulations. Examples of questions and model answers, helpful hints, together with the complete syllabus and suggested reading list mean that this book should be at the top of any candidate's shopping list. Covers both Part 1 and Part 2 examinations.

1-900364-28-X	60 pages	Published 2000